Death and Taxes

A physician's experience with the US healthcare system

Prolog	Page 3
Premed	Page 5
Medical School	Page 13
Internship and Residency	Page 40
Hanging Out Your Shingle	Page 57
Finding Patients and Building Your Practice	Page 66
Getting Paid	Page 70
How Much Do Doctors Make?	Page 83
A Day In The Life	Page 87
Family and Friends	Page 95
Playing Well With Others	Page 101
The Digital Age	Page 106
Malpractice	Page 113
Paying For It	Page 122
Selected Patient Care Issues	Page 129
Retirement	Page 152
Death and Taxes	Page 156
Epilog	Page 162

About the Author .... Page 164

Prolog

"Kirk, why did you decide to become a doctor?" I get that question quite often as I meet new people and I am getting to know them. You would think that there is a simple answer, but not so! Sometimes I think that the answer is lost in the mists of distant memory, maybe even relegated to the class of memory that might be labeled "personal myths/fables". To be frank, I can't really remember any one particular reason that propelled me into the profession of medicine. Of course I would like to think that I was led by a desire to "help other people" which is an often cited reason why people go into the medical profession. As noble as that sounds, I don't think that it was my motivation. I believe I had some sense of altruism in my young adult heart, but I think that I can properly say that "helping others" was not my motivation to pursue a medical career. I might have considered "helping" as a worthy by product of the practice of medicine, but that was about as far as I think it went in my thought processes. My prior experience with "helping" others consisted of an LDS Church mission in which I was striving to help others in a spiritual journey to find a new gospel and a new church. That was fulfilling when I was able to shepherd others to find something that brought them joy and happiness, but never in that experience did I feel like I wanted to spend my working professional life in such an endeavor. So, no I didn't go into the profession of medicine to "help others".

I might be led to answer that question by saying: "My father/other close relative was a doctor and I want to be like him/them". I had lots of medical school class mates that had that as their reason. They had watched their close relative work their lives in the medical profession and they saw something in that close proximity to the medical career that appealed to them. Maybe it was the money, maybe it was the prestige, maybe it was the public accolades a doctor receives, maybe it was that their father told them that they were going to be a doctor! Maybe the venerable family tradition was being a doctor? I know many medical families like this. But for me that was not the case. No one in my family that I ever knew had been a doctor. I later found out that my grandfather's half-brother who I never knew was a family doctor but that was nothing to me. The closest I came to this was my uncle-- my father's youngest brother-- who lived with us for a time while attending college. He was in "pre-med" planning to become a doctor when he was stricken with some health problems that led his doctor to advise him against a career in medicine because the stress of it would be bad for his health. He was disappointed to be sure, but changed his major and became a medical lab technologist. I was really close to this uncle and identified with him in many ways so I think in my young mind that may have been the first time I thought that maybe I should be a physician. Later, in my late teen years I spent a summer's month with him and accompanied him on his work at the hospital and there had my first real exposures to what medicine was all about as a profession. He worked in a small hospital and was the lab tech, the x-ray tech, and drew most of the blood specimens. He had interaction on the hospital ward and in the emergency room with the attending doctors in that small town, and I was able to observe them in the practice of their profession. That did attract me, I must say. When I started college at Brigham Young University I majored in chemistry with the intention of riding that major to medical school, but soon found out that my chemistry aptitude stopped at the graduation ceremony from high school and was not up to the rigors of the university study of that science! I wandered around through a zoology course or two, but was turned off severely by "comparative vertebrate anatomy" and lost my way, and with it my interest in medicine for a time. After returning from my church mission I was afloat without direction and after a year ended up on a track to have a major in sociology which interested me greatly. But being a university professor wasn't what I wanted to be and in the end I came back to the idea of pursuing medical school sort of on the basis that I didn't have any better idea at the time!

So, maybe the most honest answer that I can give to the question of why I decided to become a doctor is: "Well, it seemed like the thing to do at the time!" Several of my professors at BYU felt that I would make a good sociologist and offered to help me get into a good graduate program to put me on that track, but I told them I would get back to them on that if I didn't gain admission to medical school. Fortunately for me, I was able to get good grades in my major of sociology and also in the usual pre-med required courses, and even more fortunately there was a trend at the time of admitting students to medical school with more liberal and not hard science college degrees and miracle of miracles I was accepted into the University of Utah Medical school class of 1973! So, by that providence I began my study of the science and art of medicine that spanned from 1973 until I retired from active medical practice in 2015.

As it turned out, I was well suited academically, and personally for the practice of medicine. The course of study in medical school was interesting and focused on what a doctor needed to know rather than on an exhaustive study of a particular field of science. Everything seemed relevant to what I was trying to become. It turned out that I liked working with sick people (except "mental" cases—more on that later on), especially when what I did helped them to be less sick, or even to get well. Blood and gore was not pleasant but it didn't turn me off to the "icky" parts of medical practice. I discovered that I could stick needles into other people without being squeamish about it. Even cutting people with scalpels was fascinating in its own morbid way! I found that I had aptitude for diagnosis and for remembering treatments including drug names and doses. I could even spell almost all of the medical words I had to know! Somehow, the details of diseases and their manifestations found a comfortable and retrievable place in my brain. So I became a doctor in 1977 after graduating from medical school, and the rest is history.

This book is about my experiences in the practice of medicine. More than that it is about the evolution of medical practice in the United States as I experienced it in my practice. I want to herein discuss the transformation of the practice of medicine as it has occurred over that interval and to make comment about how I felt about the many changes that occurred. I also want to make comment about how I feel about where the practice of medicine is going into the future. This book then becomes not so much my memoirs of things that happened to the patients I treated, but about what happened to me as I was part of the process. Hopefully it will be a cathartic retrospective for me and more hopefully a reasoned commentary about the changes that are coming to the profession of medicine in the near future.

I chose to name this monograph "Death and Taxes" because there are not two more distinguishing characteristics of the practice of medicine than: (1) We all die! No matter how advanced medical science becomes, no matter how miraculous the medical treatments seem, no matter the breakthroughs in science and technology it still happens that we all will succumb to this terminal diagnosis that we share in common---mortality; and (2) Medicine as a general part of our economy is exorbitantly expensive and increasingly is paid for by taxing the population of the United States— "taxes". These two factors: our universal mortality and the need to fund the cost of medical care are arguably the most prominent aspects of the practice of medicine in our modern world. I have seen both factors change and evolve in the last four decades of my life in medicine and I will write about my experience and thoughts on the subject in the following chapters.

Pre-Med

So it takes a long time to become a physician. Generally speaking, a doctor has had at least four years of college education resulting in some sort of "bachelor's" degree, then another four years in medical school learning the art and science of medicine, and finally three to nine additional years learning the skills of a particular medical specialty or area of practice. All in all, a minimum of eleven years and a maximum of fifteen years past high school graduation! That makes the minimum age for a physician starting his medical practice to be about 30 years old if he or she didn't take time off to work for a while, or explored any other educational experiences other than just focusing on becoming a doctor. The time commitment to qualify for a career in medicine represents an extended time of "delayed gratification" and is a significant sacrifice made by those who pursue a medical profession. More on this later.

The time in college for the first four years has traditionally been known as "pre-med". The usual route followed has been to major in some science area such as zoology, or physiology, or math or science of some sort. Along the way most medical schools require some classes in biochemistry, physics, math and zoology. Some universities have a pre-med track with prescribed classes to take and counselors who help guide the student through the process of qualifying to apply for medical school admission. There is not however any "premed" major and you can't get a bachelor's degree in premed...what would you do with it anyway if you didn't end up getting admitted to medical school? I always advise young people who ask me to get a degree in something that interests them or that would qualify them for employment if their medical school dreams fade or are not realized. Along the way it would be helpful, even required, for the prospective doctor to have had some experience with the field of medicine by some volunteer time observing or working in some area that exposes them to medical careers. Watching TV shows about doctors just doesn't give a realistic portrayal of what it is like to actually be a doctor! Most of the pre-med students take the same classes so there is natural academic competition to do well in each class to make your application stand out to the medical school selection committee. There has been thought by some that medical students are too focused on the "hard" sciences and so some medical schools have been giving more consideration to students that had bachelor's programs in liberal arts and non-science areas thinking that they might make more humane and well-rounded doctors. I don't know if there is any data that supports this conclusion, but it is on that basis that I somehow found admission to medical school with a degree in sociology and psychology. From my perspective, I don't think I lost anything missing out on all that "hard" science in my bachelor's program since in medical school they teach you all the basic hard science you need to know to be a doctor. My medical school class had about 25% students from non-traditional pre-med undergraduate programs including myself and others with degrees in history, music, English, education, and others. Also, over the years the proportion of ethnic minority and female students has been increasing so that now 50% or more of medical school classes come from these groups. It is becoming a bit harder nowadays for your average white, middle class, Caucasian male college student to get a seat in medical school. The demographics of the medical doctors practicing in the United States has undergone a substantial shift away from white, Anglo-Saxon males in the last 40 years and continues on that course for the foreseeable future. The hope of course is that those doctors from minority ethnic groups will go back and practice medicine among their ethnic cohorts and especially in underserved areas but the reality has not matched the hope and many doctors do not return to their "roots" to practice. We in the United States still have areas of significant underservice by the medical profession. I am not advocating going back to all white Anglo-Saxon male physicians, but if our national value is to put more doctors in the underserved areas of our country we need to rethink the strategy that has been in place so far to accomplish that feat.

Other than doing well academically in their undergraduate field of study, and taking all the requisite "pre-med" courses, a prospective medical student must have stellar grades, outstanding personal recommendations from professors and other professionals who may have mentored them, and must be able to present themselves in a positive light when invited to interview at the prospective medical school by the faculty of that institution. They must also score well on the "MCAT" (Medical College Aptitude Test). This makes for a very unique set of characteristics that represent the identity of the entering medical student. They are smart, self-motivated, hard-working, self-sacrificing, high-achieving and competitive people and even the least of them are part of the top ranks of the young adults in our society. In our present world, where the rigors of entering into the practice of medicine are high and the financial opportunities to make very nice incomes are increasingly available in high tech or business careers and where the rigors and demands of a medical career are decreasingly attractive there is a declining candidate pool desiring to enter medical school. I have been unable to find reliable historical data about the ratio of applicants to admitted students for medical school but currently there are about four applicants for every medical school seat available. My impression is that there is a decreasing number of students who are interested in a medical career and that the ratio of applicants to accepted students has been falling over the last few decades. A medical career is just not as attractive in today's world to the smart young person as it once was. Less native United States students are applying to medical schools and there is an increase in foreign born students. Additionally, affirmative action laws and regulations are changing the profile of the average US medical student to more minorities, foreign born persons and women. This is good for the sake of diversity, but may not be so great for the quality of medical practitioners that are to be produced in the future. Time will be the judge of that.

Nowadays, the cost of an undergraduate degree can easily be $100,000 or more so the pre-med student unless he is well funded by some source can easily start out in medical school with substantial debt. Most undergraduate programs allow for enough time for part time employment and a social life of sorts, but that all goes away in medical school. Medical school tuition is more expensive than undergraduate with the current average medical school tuition and fees of $51,000 per year for a total of over $200,000 for the full four-year program. That puts the total cost of achieving an "MD" at over $300,000. (If the medical student goes to a Caribbean medical school—often called "off shore" schools-- the total cost for medical school alone is closer to $300,000! There are now some for-profit medical schools opening in the United States with total costs that will be similar to "off shore" medical schools. A student who pursues a medical degree in these programs could easily end up with educational debt approaching $400,000!) During medical school the course work and clinical work is so rigorous that there is little chance for part time work to help pay for things. There are very few scholarships and grants for medical students, so most go into debt for their education. The average medical school student debt is about $170,000 at the end of their medical school education and that doesn't include any residual debt carried into medical school from the undergraduate years. It is very easy for a medical student in today's world to graduate with their "MD" at a total accumulated debt of $250,000. The average medical school debt (not including undergraduate debt) in 2014 was $180,000 (according to U.S. News and World Report 5/19/2015.) If you calculate the cost of paying for that debt of $250,000 the total cost (principle plus interest) of an average medical school "MD" degree at about $332,859, or $1,849 per month (if paid at 4% over 15 years.) So you have doctors with average ages in the low 30's at the start of their practices starting out with a one third of a million dollars of debt overhead and it doesn't take a genius to understand why the number of students per medical school seat is dropping. There could easily come a time when we as a society will need to pay students to become doctors, or settle for a very different personal profile of our future doctors than we have had in the past. Especially today in the era of governmental and private insurance pressure to reduce medical costs with a large focus on reducing physician payment levels, we are going to reap a harvest of severely dropping interest in our "best and brightest" youth of entering medicine as a profession of choice. Physicians of the future will likely still earn a nice and comfortable income (although less than in the near past), but the cost of getting educated and trained may become overly burdensome especially when compared with other career tracks that take less time and money to qualify for. The motivation for our bright young people to become physicians is already in recession and will likely worsen in the next few decades. The story is told of a neurosurgeon who had a plumbing problem at his home and called for a plumber. The plumber promptly diagnosed and fixed the problem and presented the neurosurgeon with a bill of over $1000. "Wow" said the neurosurgeon, "I don't make that kind of money and I'm a neurosurgeon!" "Yeah, I know" said the plumber "I used to be a neurosurgeon too!" The point of this little vignette is that there are other ways to make the "big bucks" rather than going to all the time and expense to be a physician. Many of our best and brightest youth of the current generation are opting for less time and money intensive professions. They are choosing life-style over income. Who will be our doctors in the future?

My take on all of this is that there is need for some fundamental changes in the education of our future physician corps. The requirement for a full bachelor's degree as a pre-requisite should be seriously reexamined. A fast track undergraduate program taking two instead of four years should be considered. This would require some student profiling in high school to allow for identification of potential medical school candidates at an early time of their life. This of course would upset the US standard of a free and standardized public educational program. Some financial incentives will certainly be needed to attract the best students to the medical profession. This will require state or federal grants and scholarships to help reduce the financial burden of a medical education. This will increase the public cost of producing a medical work force. There should be adjustments in the required post MD training requirements for some medical and surgical specialties to reduce the time it takes after medical school to be qualified to practice one of the medical specialties, especially the surgical specialties. All of this will cost the public money and there is no current evidence that we will end up with an equivalent result in the quality of the medical practitioners that are produced. Also, a program such as above would result in physicians being younger ages when they start their medical practices. We as a society will have to decide whether or not we are ready to accept care from 28-year-old neurosurgeons or heart surgeons! Do adults this young have the maturity to literally hold your heart or brain in their hands? All of this represents a major paradigm shift in medical education and will be resisted by many powerful interest groups in our society not the least of which will be public education, colleges and universities and medical schools. Time will tell if that can happen, but without some changes in how we make doctors we will not be able to count on the motivated bright young adults in our society choosing medicine over a host of other less time and cost intensive occupations.

Would I tell my children or close friends to enter the medical profession? That is a hard question and I will probably answer it before the end of this monograph but my response is still formulating. The one piece of advice that I always give to any young person who asks me for my wisdom about pursuing a medical career is: "Marry someone with a rich Daddy!"

Medical School

Medical school is intense. It occupies 100 hours per week or more of the student's time. Class time and library time can easily occupy 18 hours a day including weekends. It is not for the lazy or questionably motivated student. It starts out fast accelerates. There is no medical school "101" and from day one the teaching and reading and studying schedule is full speed ahead and damn the torpedoes! It is a very focused educational program but the field of medicine is very broad so even a focused program is informationally intensive. The text books are big and written in a small font, and there are minimal pictures—what pictures are present are fully loaded with concentrated data to memorize. It is like taking a drink from a fire hose. It is very competitive with students that are highly motivated and extremely smart. Post graduate training opportunities at the most prestigious hospitals are determined in large part by class ranking and performance on nationally standardized testing. There is no time to "ease into" medical studies and the student who gets a slow start will be forever behind.

But, as intense and challenging as medical school is, the motivation of the schools is to graduate every student after four years with their "M.D." degree. Because there are limited numbers of medical school seats, and because the need for a continuing supply of doctors is high, it is in the national interest to have every first year medical student finish medical school successfully. That is even more so in our time since the 75 million strong "baby boomer generation" is just now entering the 6th decade of age—and the need for medical care really starts in this age group and continues on to the end of life. In fact, there is a deficiency between the number of doctors in training and the number of doctors needed for the coming few decades. (Current estimates put the number of physicians that we are "short" of at over 60,000 for the United States. This number is projected to be 90,000 by 2025 as reported in the Washington Post 3/3/2015.) Only in very recent years have the number of medical school seats been increased, and the number of new medical schools is minimal compared to the projected need for doctors. (According to Becker's Hospital Review 1/4/2016, 35 new medical schools were slated to open in 2015. If each produced 100 doctors per year this would produce 31,500 new doctors by 2025 compared to the need of 90,000.)

This deficiency is currently being filled with an increasing number of what have been described as "physician extenders": advance practice nurse practitioners (NP) and physician's assistants (PA). More and more in today's world, when you go to see a new doctor it is likely that you will see the NP or the PA who works for that doctor. This is not entirely satisfactory since even the best NP or PA does not have the training or experience of the marginally well trained MD (my apologies to all my NP and PA friends without which I could not have successfully practiced for the last 15 years of my professional life). But, the realities are that there are not enough doctors nationwide to service the medical needs of the population. This trend is also at least partially responsible for the increasing number of foreign born and trained physicians in the United States. Generation "X" sometimes known as the "millennials" exceeds the size of the "baby boomer" generation by about a million in large part because of the immigration of large numbers of young people into the US. The need for an expanded physician corps will continue into the foreseeable future. Where are we going to get the medical manpower to meet this need? According to a report from the Association of American Medical Colleges published April 5, 2016 (www.aamc.org) it is predicted that there will be a shortage of between 61,700 and 94,700 physicians in the next decade including shortages of both primary care physicians and specialists including surgical specialists. Whatever the solution to meeting the increasing need for medical practitioners there will be side effects and unintended consequences that cannot be foreseen and the geometrics of medical care will be very different and unpredictable in the future.

Medical school year one

The first year of the traditional medical school curriculum consists of basic science teaching. Gross anatomy, physiology, biochemistry, microbiology, pathology, medical terminology, neuroanatomy and neurophysiology, pharmacology. Just learning how to talk "med-speak" is a big part of the first year of studies. These are not exhaustive courses—each area of study has its own PhD holders and often the subjects are taught by PhD's rather than MDs. But the intent is to give the medical student enough of the basic science that medicine is based upon to have a working understanding. The first year especially is just full of large and heavy textbooks and memorization. Each subject is an "executive summary" as it were of the field. This is truly drinking from a fire hose set to high pressure! You just have to keep swallowing and try to get a breath in when you can.

The most memorable course for most of us was the gross anatomy course. We were on the first day introduced to our cadaver which we shared with a few other medical students and whom we would over the first year dissect in minute detail. For most of us this is the first experience with a dead body. (By the way, the predominant use of bodies that people "donate to science" is in gross anatomy labs, or sometimes as test "dummies" for crash tests and the like—for an interesting read on this subject see the book *Stiff: The Curious Lives of Human Cadavers* by Mary Roach). I remember passing through a doorway into the anatomy lab and there was a large vat—kind of like a large hot tub in size—which was full of formalin and had multiple cadavers floating in it…. now that was a site for innocent eyes! My cadaver was a Chinaman who had died of tuberculosis. It took some getting used to for us to stand at the table for a few hours a day and under the direction of our instructor cut away layer upon layer of the flesh of the cadaver so as to see the gross structures. Formalin smells peculiar and it is hard to get the smell of it out of your nose and clothes. Spouses and families could experience the aroma when you came home! But after a time all of us got used to it and could eat our lunches while happily dissecting away on some limb or organ. In retrospect I think the whole purpose was to desensitize us to the human body and to help us come to view it with scientific dispassion. Our gross anatomy instructor was Edward Hashimoto M.D. who was a delightful Japanese physician and who had the wonderful talent of being able to draw simultaneously with both hands with colored chalk on the black board illustrations of the anatomy we were supposed to be learning. Every few weeks we would be tested on our knowledge by going from table to table and identifying different labeled structures from all of the cadavers in the lab. The practical use of all of this knowledge finds it's expression in two main medical specialties: surgery and radiology/imaging. Now-a-days people can be virtually dissected by ultrasound, CT scanning and MRI scanning that has been a boon for diagnosis and to direct surgical treatments. Almost never is there a need to do "exploratory" surgery to make a diagnosis anymore since the imaging technology is now advanced enough to see even the tiniest anatomic structures in detail. But despite the fact that detailed images can now be obtained in living individuals, the tradition of gross anatomy lab in medical school continues. May it ever be thus!

Medical school year two

The second year of medical school is traditionally spent learning about diseases. This is usually taught in an organ system approach—i.e. cardiac diseases, pulmonary diseases, infectious diseases, etc. This is a very broad field and most of these individual diseases have medical specialists who become expert in the diagnosis and treatment of various pieces and parts of our bodies. Despite that, the medical student is expected to become familiar with all of the diseases and be able to recite signs and symptoms and basic treatments for them all. In this year the caliber of the fire hose increases by a factor of 10! There is no time to linger over one system's diseases because the next system is on the schedule with only an examination about your knowledge of the previous system to separate them in time. Eighteen hours a day is really not sufficient and mental fatigue sets in fast and often. But it is fascinating stuff and the student is starting to get a fund of knowledge that he came to medical school to obtain. The lab portion of the second year of study is experience with actual living patients. The basics of taking a medical history and of doing a physical exam are taught by practicing on real living people...including your fellow medical students, and including willing friends, spouses and other family members! You learn which end of the stethoscope goes in your ears, how to take a proper blood pressure, how to examine different body parts, and how to assess normal from abnormal anatomy and function. With all of this study of anatomy and diseases you end up looking at people you pass in the mall or on the street with a very different perspective than you did before medical school. People start to become perceived as patients and you just can't help yourself from rendering a silent medical diagnosis to random people who you see in public places! Learning "differential diagnosis" which is the process of formulating a list of possible diseases that may explain the individual patient's symptoms and physical exam findings is emphasized. With the highly motivated, excessively compulsive medical student this can sometime lead to some humorous events. I will describe two:

I remember being assigned a woman to interview and examine and come back with a differential diagnosis. I was nervous of course and wanted to be sure I didn't miss asking a single question or examining even the smallest part of her anatomy. Being unsure of myself I would take copious notes and make notation after each question or examination. I remember that I thought I had obtained a complete history of every possible medical point that applied to her. Then I was into the examination phase. As I pulled down her gown to listen to her heart and lungs I could not identify any breasts! I was sure she had not had a mastectomy so what could this mean? I rechecked my notes—sure enough no mention of mastectomies. I even asked her directly at that moment whether or not she had had mastectomies. Well, the mystery was solved when I pulled up her gown to examine her abdomen and found two very droopy breasts lying just above her groin area! Well I was simultaneously relieved, amazed and grossed out all at the same time. She was understanding, bless her heart.

We were taught how to do pap smears by each practicing on "models" that were hired by the medical school. (It was our opinion that these women were probably of ill repute so to speak. I don't know if that was true or not.) Imagine each of 4 or 5 models having a clumsily performed pap smear 20 or more times by inexperienced and embarrassed medical students. Well, one of our class mates was so nervous he kept getting in the back of the line until he was the very last one to have the pap smear experience. Well, he walks in trying not to look the woman in the face when she rises up on an elbow and says: "Rich, Hi, do you remember me?" (I think a former high school classmate.) Rich immediately responded by fainting dead out on the floor. This was such a memorable event in our class that it was reenacted during our post-graduation party. But, the end of the story is just as funny—Rich became an obstetrician/gynecologist!

During the second year studies many of us recognized symptoms of the diseases that we were studying in ourselves. If you had even the slightest bit of hypochondria this was a hazard because you started to believe that you had this or that horrendous disease! Paranoia ran a bit rampant as many of my classmates took the professors aside to discuss their personal symptoms and to find out if they were dying from the disease of the day! But it was not so funny with one of my classmates who thought that his spleen might be enlarged and in fact it was and he was subsequently diagnosed with lymphoma. He subsequently had surgery to remove the spleen and had complications of that surgery that led to his death. That was all the more personal to me because this particular classmate was the son of one of the physicians that I had come to know and like while I was accompanying my uncle Terry during a summer in Richfield, Utah so many years before. Since then, it has become my experience that us physicians are very poor at recognizing disease in ourselves. Most of the times we ignore obvious symptoms either because we are too busy or more often because of self-deception and denial. This leads many physicians to postpone diagnosis of their own personal medical problems until late into the disease process. Physicians die at a faster and earlier age than many of their age matched peers and I think it may be because through the course of our training and practice we learn to not see ourselves in the diseased patients that we treat. We thus ignore symptoms that any second year medical student would recognize dismissing them as "second year syndrome". While on this topic I will here confess that I never liked taking care of another physician or their wives because they were terrible patients! They would often miss follow up appointments, would often be non-compliant with tests ordered or treatments prescribed, tended to substitute their own "prescriptions" for treatment with the one that I had recommended, or refused to take my diagnosis no matter how fully documented it was. I will here also confess that I personally fit the profile I just described! The counsel "physician heal thyself" is poor advice however and a long held medical truth is that "the physician who treats himself has a fool for a patient" is proved true way too often.

    At the end of the second year of medical school the student must take part one of the National Board of Medical Examiners test for medical students. This is a two-part test—part one at the end of the second year of medical school and part two at the end of the fourth year of medical school. Both parts are exhaustive multiple choice tests, 2 days of examination each, with hundreds of questions that can and do come from every topic studied in the first two years of medical school. The tests are timed and questions that are not answered are counted against your final score. Needless to say, it is an intimidating experience. A medical student must pass both parts of the exam after completion of medical school to be eligible for a medical license. Well, as fate would have it my wife was pregnant with our third child and was due to deliver a few weeks after the part one testing date. I repeatedly told her that under no circumstances was she to deliver our child during the examination---well sure I jinxed it! After I came exhausted home from day one of the exam my wife was looking a bit iffy, but we both felt that maybe if we just got some sleep we would both be ok. We got the other two children in bed and were ready to settle in ourselves when she told me that she was quite sure that she was in labor! I reassured her with all of my obstetrics knowledge (which equaled "none") that she was not in labor and just go to sleep. That might have sufficed except her water broke and then we knew for sure how poor of an obstetrical diagnostician I was! So off to the hospital we went, and our son was born very late that night or early that next morning depending upon how you want to quantify the night. I got no sleep, arrived home only in time to settle the children with a neighbor, take a shower and eat a hasty breakfast, and then off for day two of the exam. But God blessed me, or I guessed well (it was a "multiple guess" formatted test), and thanks to the stimulant action of Coca Cola I was able to get through the second day of testing with a passing grade. While on the topic of Coca Cola I will here state that the medical profession runs on caffeine! Either in the form of coffee or caffeinated beverages it is the same. The schedule of medical school starts it out, but to keep up a medical practice with 50 to 60 hours work per week, nights spent interrupted by phone calls and trips to the hospital, and any attempt to live some sort of "normal" non-medical life leaves almost every physician sleep deprived. If it weren't for caffeine this all would be impossible. Never begrudge your doctor his caffeine.

As I mentioned before, medical students are bright, obsessive, and competitive. At the end of the second year of study the top students are inducted into the AOA (Alpha Omega Alpha) which is the honor society for medical students. It is a prestigious honor society and often is the first medical school credential that offers placement into the best post graduate training programs. I wasn't inducted! Oh well, you didn't need to be a member of AOA to be a good physician—that's what we all told ourselves, and in reality it is true. I do remember one member of our class who was inducted into AOA telling us all at the time of graduation that: "I have forgotten more than any of the rest of you learned!" and he meant it. It was likely true also, but so what? To be a good doctor you have to be continually learning and studying even during your practice years. There is no body of knowledge that can be learned in medical school that will suffice for a 30 to 40-year practice lifetime. Continuing medical education (CME) is essential to keep up with the fast pace of medical science and treatments. CME is required yearly for renewal of a doctor's medical license. But the CME has become an industry in itself with expensive "courses" offered at exotic locations (can you say "Hawaii", "Las Vegas", and others) and at high cost. There was a time when drug companies offered CME at their expense often on cruise ships or other resort locations, laced very heavily with promotion of their company's current "wonder drugs." Most of these self-promoting CME adventures are now banned, but for a time doctors got wonderful free vacations with some CME attached. Even now, there are doctors who make big bucks on the traveling lecture circuit sponsored by drug companies doing CME to physicians and hospitals. You have heard of the military-industrial complex for sure that seems to produce $500 toilet seats and the like, well, there is a very real CME-medical complex that injects capitalistic self interest in the continuing education of physicians. As an alternative to of all of this there is very affordable CME available now and most physicians, while being compulsive, and motivated to be the best they can be are also socially responsible and are opting out of the abusive CME-medical complex and choosing instead more socially responsible forms of CME. One thing for sure is that if a doctor quits learning and improving his medical skills he becomes a hazard to his community of patients. Rules have been passed now and the most that a physician may expect to "get" from a drug company representative may be lunch or maybe a free pen or some sticky note pads with the latest miracle drug name emblazoned upon it.

Just to give you a taste of the pace of medical science and how much it is necessary for a physician to continue learning both knowledge and skills as he pursues his medical practice career I will give a few examples. When I was in medical school the treatment for stomach ulcers was a bland diet and 7 doses per day of an antacid liquid. Surgery was often done for ulcers that failed that regimen. At the end of my medical school time a miracle drug for ulcers came out—Tagamet—which changed dramatically the treatment success for ulcer patients. Since then whole new classes of acid suppressing medications have been developed each with different doses, effectiveness, and side effects. On top of that a bacterium known as helicobacter pylori was discovered that was found to be responsible for a large majority of ulcer disease and is curable with a program of antibiotics. Surgery for ulcer patients is a very rare thing now. None of that was known when I was in my medical school training. Antibiotics have exploded in number and effectiveness. When I was in medical school there were only a few different classes of antibiotics. Now the number is mind-numbing. Not only that, as antibiotics have become more used—and over used—bacteria have learned how to be resistant to them. There are now starting to arise in the world strains of pathological bacteria that are resistant to all the currently available antibiotics. Once infection was the number one killer of people, then antibiotics changed that, but now with the emergence of antibiotic resistant bacteria we can't be sure that the "bugs" might not win the survival battle with humans in the end. A physician has to keep up with the medical literature to keep abreast of this rapidly changing balance between antibiotics and bacteria. The amount of paper in the hundreds of medical journals and publications kills unknown numbers of trees yearly! When I was in medical school coronary artery bypass grafting for coronary disease was only a decade old at best and still not widely available in the United States. Of course, now cardiac surgeons do it routinely and even do heart transplants and other miraculous surgeries. But the cardiologists have developed many catheter-delivered heart treatments that replace the need for coronary bypass grafting and even some valve replacements can now be done via a catheter. Prevention of coronary disease with medications including "statins" and other drugs is a rapidly changing field. Surgery used to involve big incisions and large scars, but the development of "scope" assisted surgery has changed the face of surgery of about every body part. There were no CT scans then and MRI was several decades after I graduated from medical school. None of these and many other examples were known or taught in medical school in my era. Without putting in serious and consistent effort to keep pace with the expansion of medical and surgical science, a physician could quickly become incompetent. An adage of medical practice has and continues to be: "never be the first to use a new treatment…. nor the last!" A good physician stays up to date but does not experiment upon their patients with the newest thing until it is well established to be both safe and effective. It is a serious challenge to be up to date in your specialty but most physicians that I know make a serious effort to do so.

Medical school year three

The third and fourth years of medical school are involved with the clinical care of patients. Most of the time is spent in the hospital or in medical clinics and there is no further formal classroom teaching. It is up to the student to learn the art and science of medicine by personal study, and by observation and participation in the care of actual patients. In that regard the educational theme of these clinical years is: "See one, do one, teach one" (more on that below). Medical students are assigned in turn to the major hospital "services" –these are the different medical departments including surgery, medicine, pediatrics, neurology, psychiatry, OB-Gynecology and the like. The third year is involved in rotation through each of these main specialty areas of medicine and the fourth year allows for experience is some of the subspecialty areas like ENT, Urology, Gastroenterology, Cardiology, Rehab, etc. The fourth year allows the medical student options to have experience in medical specialty areas and is often used to get exposure to an area of practice that the student may want to pursue as his medical career or to become known to a specialty physician who may be willing to give a recommendation to a post graduate training program that the student may want to get into after graduation. In this regard, the medical student who knows "what they want to be when they grow up" is at a distinct advantage. I had many classmates that from day one knew they wanted to be an ophthalmologist, or an orthopedic surgeon, or such and so their choices of the fourth year were geared to make that happen. To medical students like myself who didn't know what they wanted to be, it was an opportunity to test out what practicing in these specialty areas might be like in reality. I started out in medical school thinking I wanted to be a pediatrician although the reasons for that are lost in the fog of ancient memory. But I found out when on my pediatric "rotation" that taking care of small persons who couldn't talk and only cried to voice their symptoms was not for me! Likewise, I found no passion in delivering babies, and surgery made my hand eczema flare up from the frequent scrubbing before surgery. (And besides, I had worked my way through my undergraduate degree at BYU cutting meat in the meat department and didn't think I would have much luck recruiting patients as a surgeon if they found out that I had worked my way through school as a butcher!) I did find out however that I liked taking care of adults in the hospital and the field of internal medicine became my career choice by default! More on that in a later chapter.

So, in the third year for most medical students we transition through the major divisions of medicine: surgery, internal medicine, pediatrics, OB-GYN, and psychiatry. You as the medical student become part of a team made up of an attending physician (a real honest to goodness practicing doctor!), a resident physician who is an MD who is working his way through the training process to become a physician in that particular specialty, an intern who is an MD in their first year of post MD training and may or may not be planning to continue on into additional training in this particular field, and a medical student. Each patient then ends up getting interviewed and examined by each member of the team often starting with the medical student, then the intern, then the resident and finally by the attending doctor. This allows for supervised learning of the art and science of that particular branch of medicine. Unfortunately, it exposes the poor patient to being asked many of the same questions and examined in much the same manner by 4 different practitioners. You know the old adage about "stuff generally runs downhill"—well that is true here and the most mundane and tedious aspects of the medical care are relegated to the lower levels in the team. So the poor medical student gets stuck with doing the stuff that no one else wants to do, while the more complicated and technical aspects of the care are done by the higher level physicians. But the general pattern of "see one, do one, teach one" is the mode of learning. Each of the basic medical skills is first demonstrated to the medical student, then done by the medical student with supervision, and then the medical student usually in the 4th year or internship year teaches the procedure to the newest members of the team. That is why you don't want to be a patient in a teaching hospital from June through September (maybe even later) of any year because June is the usual time that new interns and residents start their rotations and the patient is subjected to the care of inexperienced physicians. Of course the attending physician is in theory present to supervise the care rendered by the new doctors, but that is at best a supposition, and at worst an exaggeration. And, the interns and the residents are the first physicians on call to respond to changes in the patient's condition or to emergencies. "See one, do one, teach one" results in some mistakes being made, but is the only way to put the new medical student and the new doctor in a position where they are forced in real time to learn the skills of a competent physician. When it works the way it should there is always backup by a more experienced physician, but the ideal is not always realized. So, try not to get sick during those months, at least not sick enough to land in the hospital! Honestly, I just don't see how the system could be changed and still allow for the critical real time decision making experiences that a new physician needs to make to learn the art of his craft. The myth that seems to be promoted by all the "Doctor" TV shows of doctors who know everything, have done everything, and think totally clearly and fast on their feet is just not reality. The reality is that you are not sure what to do, you have to look up doses of medications to be sure you got them right, you need to consult with your senior members on the team, and all the while the patient is sick and needing treatment. In the ideal world all patients in the hospital would be taken care of by only experienced and knowledgeable physicians who have been in practice for years and know both the science and art of medicine. That reality is most closely met in the non-teaching hospitals (those hospitals that don't have medical students, interns or residents), but even there more and more the hospital care of patients is done by "hospitalists" who are in general young, newly out of their training programs, and less than well-seasoned physicians—more about that in another chapter.

My first clinical rotation as a medical student was on the psychiatric ward. Up to that time I had never known anybody that I thought was mentally ill. I had a few anxious family members with depressive tendencies but none were "crazy" to use a term. I was totally naive. The first patient that was assigned to me was a middle aged paranoid schizophrenic woman who's paranoia was focused on the delusion that her husband was spying on her all the time. He could take many shapes and forms and faces and could even see her through the TV and radio. I was doing pretty well though I thought until about half an hour into the interview when she paused and then looked straight into my eyes and said: "You are my husband, aren't you?" I was freaked! Somehow I stumbled through the rest of the interview but I was shaken by the experience. Next, I was assigned to interview a 20-year-old young man who was both schizophrenic and homosexual. Now, this was in the early 1970s you have to understand and was a long time before homosexuality was as accepted as it is in our present day. As far as I knew I had never met a homosexual person. And I came from a very sexually repressed heritage in which the word "sex" was rarely uttered and never talked about or explained. Well, this young man had been discharged from service in his church as a missionary when he had the psychotic break, and only when that happened did his homosexuality become an open issue. Well, by noon of that day I was suffering all the signs of psychosomatic illness—I had a severe tension headache, my back and neck felt like the muscles were so tight that my back was breaking, and I was nauseated with a rock in my stomach and had no interest in lunch! Welcome to the world of psychiatry! After lunch time I was starting to feel just a little bit better when the next patient I was assigned to was a middle aged male pedophile who was court ordered in for a 30-day psychiatric evaluation. This man was despicable and I sincerely loathed him. So much for being the model of a detached medical observer who dispassionately evaluates each patient as if they were some type of scientific study without any judgement or value superimposition regarding their situation. By the end of that day I was certain that the field of psychiatry was not for me. It was not easy going back for day two. But, as with almost everything else in medicine, after six weeks of exposure to many such patients I could do my medical duties without all the psychosomatic side effects that I experienced that first day. Medical school is a series of desensitization experiences for students to help them become at ease with facing difficult patients and difficult medical situations. We must learn to be unflappable in the face of things that would cause the layman to freak out and run away screaming! No one formally teaches the student those coping skills...they are self-learned as self-defensive skills and I think some of the personality traits that physicians exhibit that are the most complained about by patients represent maladaptive learned behaviors acquired by treating difficult patients and diseases in medical school and beyond. Physicians are humans who are shaped by the experiences that they have and who adapt sometimes in dysfunctional ways. The adaptations required of the doctor make them emotionally distant, authoritative, presumptive, suspicious, and lacking in empathy for their patients. All of these character traits help the doctor maintain some semblance of sanity while dealing with patients who are demanding, noncompliant, and not at their best because of illness and also who have sometimes terrible and tragic illnesses. Unfortunately, these traits are not just a mask that the physician puts on at the beginning of their work day and takes off at night, but they become a permanent part of their personality. This results in a tendency to dysfunctional relationships even with their spouses and friends and close family.

My second clinical rotation was greatly anticipated because I entered medical school thinking that I wanted to be a pediatrician. Although I didn't have any psychosomatic reactions to taking care of sick children, I found that I was not suited to the practice of pediatrics. Two reasons: (1) Mothers who either were so involved that they were interfering, or too remote to care much at all about their child. (2) Little children are small, and they are not articulate. They tell you they are sick by crying—a universal signal for everything from a wet diaper to meningitis! I did find however the most compassionate and caring of all the doctors I trained with were the pediatricians and pediatric specialists. They were exceptional human beings and so kind and caring that I would have been happy to be numbered among them if it weren't for the fact that I just didn't like taking care of little children. As a father of little children myself, I also had a hard time emotionally finding the proper "professional detachment" from the patients that I was treating. I also had one personal experience with pediatric trauma that again proved to me that I made the right choice not to go into pediatrics. While I was doing my post graduate residency in internal medicine I accidentally backed over my 2-year-old son as I pulled the car into the garage. He suffered rib fractures, a basal skull fracture, cerebral contusions and traumatic pancreatitis and was hospitalized for about a week. Fortunately, he survived with no apparent residual problems...he is now a CPA working for a specialized financial services corporation. The doctors and nurses and pediatric staff were great all but the medical students who were so keen on seeing the blood behind my son's left ear drum (a physical finding of basal skull fracture) that he was bothered over and over again until my wife put a stop to it. Medical students are just so anxious to see everything and do everything that they sometimes forget the human element in medicine...patients are "real" people with all the emotions and needs that implies. Some doctors never get over that stage and are forever described by their patients as detached, rough, and blunt and non-caring. Medicine is described as both an art and a science. Medical school is mostly about learning the science of medicine, but along the way the art of medicine has to be learned otherwise doctors become competent scientists but incompetent human beings. The art of medicine is usually taught by example and fortunately there are many caring, compassionate and gentle doctors who mentor medical students along the way, but there are no formal classes to instruct medical students how to practice the art of medicine. The stress of practicing medicine with the need to see high volumes of patients can make even the most caring and kind physician come off as lacking empathy and understanding of the emotional toll that patients suffer because of their illnesses. Physicians are compensated financially for practicing the science of medicine and not the art so when the practicalities of earning a living practicing medicine fall upon them, most physicians practice the science of medicine at the expense of the art of medicine. Some of that also happens because a physician would have to have a remarkable depth of emotional strength to not be devastated by all the suffering that illness causes their patients, so to insulate themselves emotionally they develop a distant personality. Doctors must develop some degree of emotional detached from their patient's distress just for self-preservation. In my case, I found that I was not successfully able to find that "right amount" of detachment from pediatric patients to successfully become a pediatrician. On a different note, pediatricians are perennially at or near the bottom of physician income levels. Increasingly less and less doctors are opting for a career in pediatrics because the work hours, emotional toll on the physician, and the demands of diagnosing illness in little ones who can't talk to you are just not adequately compensated with financial reward. Pediatricians more than any other doctor set I know practice their craft because they feel a "calling" to care for children. More will be said later about the inequalities of monetary compensation among the different specialties of medical practice.

My OB-GYN rotation quickly taught me that I did not want to be a deliverer of babies either! This was not much of a revelation since the practice of OB/GYN was never attractive to me in the first place. By this time in my life I had been married several years and was the father of three children so I pretty much knew where babies came from! But I did learn some valuable lessons during my time on the OB/GYN service. I was involved with the delivery of a baby with a 16-year-old mother from a lower socioeconomic class of society. I had been taught to routinely ask post-partum mothers about bodily functions post-delivery to be sure that all was getting back to normal. Thus, dutifully each morning when I saw her (moms and babies stayed in the hospital for 3-4 days after birth back in those times) I asked her about these and specifically if she had yet had a bowel movement—to which she answered "no". After a few days questioning and receiving the answer "no" I was getting a little alarmed but decided more questioning was the first order of concern. So I asked again and she responded with "what does it feel like when your bowel moves?" When I finally asked her "have you taken a crap since your baby was born?" she immediately answered "yes, right afterwards!" There is a vocabulary and language gap between doctors and patients that can lead to misunderstanding or worse. "Doctor-speak" is not like normal speech. Medical terms are not part of the usual citizen's vocabulary and when you factor that in with differences in native language it can lead to misunderstanding. It is often hard for doctors to use "normal words" to describe medical tests, treatments and diagnosis because the medical vocabulary that is learned as part of their medical training has been developed to portray a lot of information in specific technical words and phrases. Doctors know what they are talking about, but the challenge is to make patients know also. Especially in times that there are serious medical problems such as cancer, etc. doctors need to be sure that their patients not only understand, but that they have no possible misunderstanding about their medical condition. That is a skill that is variably learned by doctors in training and is not formally taught in medical school. Add to that the pressures of medical practice with the need to see many patients per day in order to be financially able to support a medical practice. The doctor is often rushed to give his advice and then rapidly move on to the next patient. Patients should not just nod and say "yes doctor" and if they do not understand what the doctor has said they should question until they clearly understand. But in the real world especially when the doctor is perceived as occupying a high social position of authority and prestige compared to the patient the patient often leaves the doctor encounter not really knowing what the diagnosis or treatment plan is. This leaves the patient unequipped to participate in their own care and often also leads to patient noncompliance with the treatment regimen due to poor understanding. It also leads to patient's perception that doctors are not caring or concerned about the effects of the illness on the patient's personal and family life. Now in our modern world with the internet so widely available patients often supplement their understanding by their own "surfing" of the web. Unfortunately, there is so much medical misinformation out there that this practice usually does nothing to improve either understanding or compliance on the part of the patient. Patients may occasionally get and read their own medical records. This is especially prone to misunderstanding because medical records are made entirely in "doctor speak" without any attempt to translate them into lay language. Miscommunication is at the root of almost all dysfunctional social interactions and has potentially life threating consequences in the doctor-patient setting. Medical care is a physician-patient combined endeavor and the best doctor is the one who can effectively and without misunderstanding inform his patient-partner about the diagnosis and treatment plan.

    General surgery is the next of the core hospital services that the medical student spends time in. To my way of thinking the surgeons were masochists! Usually the first scheduled surgery starts at 7am so rounds to see the patients in the hospital were usually started at 5 a.m. so they could be seen and problems addressed before the surgery team is in the operating room for the rest of the day. Surgery starts at 7a.m. and depending on the schedule the surgical team can be in the OR for the next 8-12 hours. The rule of thumb is that the only surgery that starts on time is the first scheduled one and that is only if something from the emergency department doesn't bump that one out of position. After the surgical team got done with the day's operations, then they needed to see that day's post-operative patients before calling it a day. So the average surgical intern and resident's days were routinely 12 to 18 hours long! Then factor in night "call" and it was easy for a medical student on a surgical team to spend 2.5 or more days straight in the hospital before any time off to go home, rest and recuperate, only to start it up again in 24 hours. Add to that the fact that the usual time spent in a surgical residency before you were ready to go out and start a surgery practice is 5 years and you might understand why the allure of a surgical career was not for me. Many of the surgical specialties like neurosurgery added another 2-3 years to that time frame so it could easily take 7 or 8 years after graduation from medical school to be able to start your surgical career. Your average surgeon is in his early thirties before he is ready to hang out his shingle and start his medical practice. But my, it could be exciting to have the routine gallbladder surgery punctuated with dramatic emergency surgeries just like you see on the popular TV doctor's shows. Surgeons are the stars of the medical profession. They get all the glory and all the girls! Their motto is: "A chance to cut is a chance to cure!" They can often be described as having an attitude that there is no disease process that cannot be cured by the application of a Bard-Parker scalpel blade. Surgeons are the doctors that do the things that allow hospitals to make a lot of money so they are highly prized members of any hospital medical staff. Unfortunately for the medical student, the experience on the surgical rotation is at least one row back from the patient's side during surgeries and all of the busy work like writing orders, pre-operative testing and assessment, and post op routine care is relegated to them. It isn't until a few years into the surgical training program that the doctor gets to take something out or put something into the patient. You must really want to be a surgeon to subject yourself to the rigors of surgical training. Surgeons as a general rule make at least 50 to 100% more than non-operating specialists (this rule is broken by radiologists who are always near the top of physician earnings) so there are real financial rewards for enduring the grueling training of a surgeon. For me, I just wasn't interested in that whole ordeal. And besides my hand eczema was severely aggravated by all the hand washing that was involved with surgery. General surgery serves as the basis for the training of all the surgical specialists so if the medical student wants to be an orthopedic surgeon or a neurosurgeon or a cardiovascular surgeon they need to do well in the surgical rotation in their third year of medical school.

The last of the third year rotations is internal medicine. This is the place where all the adult patients who aren't having surgery are taken care of in the hospital. Here the patients have many illnesses ranging from undiagnosed problems that are requiring hospitalization to solve to people with aggravation of chronic health problems such as diabetes or heart disease, to acute infections such as pneumonia, to heart attacks and strokes and any other illness that requires hospital care but will not need surgery. The field of internal medicine is very broad and includes all of the specialties that many people know about including cardiology, gastroenterology, rheumatology, oncology and many others. The medical student here gets to be part of the diagnostic and treatment team. Usually when a patient is admitted to medicine the medical student is one of the first to see the patient, followed by the intern, then the resident. At each step of the process the medical student is allowed to participate in the diagnostic work up of the patient as well as the treatment. This was very stimulating to me, and I found that taking care of sick adults was much more to my aptitude than taking care of sick children on the pediatric service. Part of the rigor for the medical student on the medicine service was to learn how to "present" a patient to the attending doctor—a mental process in which the most important symptoms, physical findings, lab and x-ray aspects of the patient's case are described to the attending physician and the rest of the team in a brief but complete narrative. Of course as part of the experience the attending doctor may ask any question of the presenter and the anxiety of the medical student (and later of the medicine intern and resident) is to have a ready answer to any and every inquiry. You had to learn to think on your feet and under pressure and to have read and studied widely enough that you could answer the questions about the patient. The culmination of this learning to "present" a patient was presenting a patient to one of the senior professors of medicine. Upon your performance in this event was based a large part of your evaluation as a medical student. In my case I was required to present the case of a patient with progressive systemic sclerosis to Dr. Maxwell Wintrobe one of the founders of the University of Utah medical school and a doctor of world-wide notoriety in his field of hematology. He was the author of one of the authoritative textbooks in his field. Dr. Wintrobe had a reputation for "chewing up and spitting out" medical students so I was anxious to say the least. I studied night and day for several days in preparation. Dr. Wintrobe was a man of diminutive stature but of regal bearing. I presented the case to him and then after giving the pertinent medical facts, described our diagnostic and treatment plan for this patient, and then followed with a short dissertation on the disease itself. Either I did a great job or Dr. Wintrobe had a long night previous to my presentation, because when all was done I was neither chewed up nor spit out! So, after finding that I didn't want to be a psychiatrist, that taking care of sick children was not what I had previously imagined, that OB/GYN held no interest for me and that surgery made my hands hurt and left me feeling like my life as a surgeon would leave no time for family and other pursuits, I was relieved to find that there might be a place for me to practice internal medicine for my career. And that children is how I came to be an Internist!

So I ended my third year of medical school with the intent of pursuing a career practicing internal medicine. As the years rolled on I found that was a good choice for me. The scientific basis for internal medicine is engaging, and the breadth of patient diagnoses treated made for a very interesting career. I also found that I related well to my patients who were in large part older people with chronic diseases. It was gratifying to me to take care of patients over a very long time so that I got to know them personally, and not just as a single medical encounter. As an internist I felt that I was qualified to be the primary physician for the bulk of adult patients, and there was a demand for my specialty. And although the practice of internal medicine is busy and demanding, I did find time to stay involved with my family and to participate in other non-medical activities.

Medical school year four

The fourth year of medical school generally involves mostly "electives"— that is we could choose from a variety of clinical experiences mostly based upon our plans for our medical careers. There were still very time intensive rotations on some of the hospital services that involved night and ER call and 16 hour days, but there were also clinic rotations working with doctors in outpatient offices seeing ambulatory patients working just daytime hours and with no "on call" demands. Up until that time all of our clinical experiences were with sick patients in the hospital, and it was revealing to see what the outpatient clinic practice of medicine was like. I took electives usually of 6 to 8 weeks' duration in cardiology, gastroenterology, rheumatology and other of the internal medicine subspecialty areas. Some of my fellow students spent time doing research with some of the professors. This year was more low key than the three previous years. There was not so much time-intensive studying, or long days and nights in the hospital. The studying was usually on problems specific to the patients that were being seen in the clinic. This was also a time to try to get to know more personally the professors that you would be asking to write letters of recommendation for post MD internship and residency programs. During this year I also found opportunities to "moonlight" for pay...the first time since entering medical school that I was to be compensated financially for some of what I had learned. I got a job doing night coverage at one of the local hospitals that did not have medical students, interns or residents. Mostly my job was to start IV's that the nurses couldn't start, and occasionally respond to a patient who developed a new fever or some other problem that the attending doctor felt comfortable with me evaluating. A lot of the time was spent reading and studying and sleeping. The other part of the time in the fourth year was spent in making application for a place to do internship and residency training. This involved a paper application process along with submitting letters of recommendation and hopefully some invitations to do on site interviews. In this process, prior performance in the first 3 years was important and things like AOA recognition and personal references from the medical school faculty doctors was important. If you had desires to get a training program appointment at one of the big time hospitals like Johns Hopkins in Baltimore, or Mass General in Boston, or Duke in South Carolina, or Stanford in California, etc. you needed to have the backing of the prominent medical faculty at the medical school you attended. This process all culminated in an event known as the "match" which took place in March of the 4th year of medical school.

The "match" is a very nervous time for medical students. The process is as follows: the medical student decided what specialty he wanted to pursue for his medical career and then made application to the hospitals of his choice that offered training in that area. The student then ranked his preference from 1 to 10 and submitted that to a centralized organization. The various hospitals that offered internships and residency training also submit their choices of medical students who had applied to them ranked 1 to 10 to the same organization. After a specified deadline for application someone at the organization pushed the "enter" key on the computer and it did what computers do and produced the appointments for the students at the various post MD training hospitals. On a specified day all the fourth year medical students met together in a big classroom and each in turn was given an envelope that was going to be their life for the next three to 7 years! Sometimes you "matched" with your first choice, and sometimes with your 10th. A few unfortunates didn't "match" at all. Sometimes all of the available slots at a particular hospital were filled, and sometimes not, so after the process there was time for individual negotiations between medical students and hospitals. Eventually all the medical students (with a very few exceptions) would find a place to move on to the next phase of their training. The medical school of course had records of where their students matched and they would crow about how many of their students got "matched" to the nationally prestigious training programs. In a way it was like a college football program making a big deal about how many of its players got drafted into the NFL! For me, I had been "promised" a position at the University of Utah by a few of the Internal

Medicine department professors and had ranked the U of U as my number one choice. But in the end I matched with LDS hospital in Salt Lake City which was my 2nd choice. After a few minutes of irritation about that I was satisfied that I had done OK...I did not have to move to a different city or state, and I was familiar with LDS hospital and some of the staff there. It wasn't a track to a career as a professor at a medical school but that was not my career plan, and so off I went to LDS hospital as an intern in June of 1977.

    A few comments are in order regarding the "match" and the career fallout from that process. First, some specialties in medicine have a limited number of training slots for interns and residents. We don't need as many neurosurgeons for instance as we need primary care doctors, and because of this there is not a large number of training slots for neurosurgeons, etc. So if you are wanting to be a radiologist, or a dermatologist, or a pathologist or a neurosurgeon or some other type of "-ologist" with limited numbers of training slots the process is at times very competitive and some medical students are denied their career choices because they can't get a training position. But there was still some hope since all states in the United States required one post MD year of training—known as the "internship"—before the new doctor could apply for and be granted a medical license to practice medicine. As with anything else at the end of the internship there were some people who changed their minds about their career plans or other things would happen that would lead to training slots opening up here and there that might give the initially disappointed young doctor another chance to become what he wanted to be when he grew up. On the flip side, there were usually more internship and residency slots open in the primary care fields—especially family practice and internal medicine, and to a lesser extent pediatrics—than there were graduates of American medical schools to fill. This resulted in many of these slots going unfilled by the "match" process for US educated medical students. Many of these slots were then filled with foreign trained medical students. The net result of all of this is that over the last 4 or 5 decades in the United States, more and more primary care track slots are being filled by foreign trained medical students and now in essentially any community of any size in the United States there are foreign born doctors taking care of the

US population. A very large proportion of these foreign born and educated medical students come from the Middle Eastern countries, and from Pakistan, China and India. So if you wonder when you go to see a doctor in any town in the USA why you will often be cared for by a doctor from one of these foreign countries, well, this is why. And since the "subspecialty" areas that are derived from Internal Medicine—cardiology, gastroenterology, pulmonology, oncology, nephrology, rheumatology, etc. are filled by those doctors who complete internal medicine training it is also true that over the last 4 to 5 decades these prestigious medical specialties are increasingly being filled with foreign born doctors. This is true also of the surgical specialties. Now I am not saying that this is a bad thing. These foreign born and medical school educated doctors are competent and caring and are providing valuable service to the US population. But, given the current trends that do not seem to be changing, it is conceivable that in another few decades essentially all the primary care doctors and a large proportion of the specialty physicians as well will be foreign born and won't have English as their native language. I will leave it to the reader to make their own conclusions about this, but it is the future! The failure of the education of medical doctors in the United States to attract and train doctors from the native United States population is an area that should be a subject of public discussion and policy just as much as the payment for medical services in the United States.

There is a natural tendency for medical students to want to become some kind of specialist or another. However, the population of the United States doesn't need large numbers of neurosurgeons etc., but it needs large numbers of primary care physicians. Specialists garner more prestige and respect than generalists. Specialists also make more money that generalists. Specialists often have more favorable personal time schedules than generalists and the dollar/hour for their work often out strips the generalist doctor by a factor of 4- 5 to 1. Because of this there is becoming an imbalance in the United States of the number of generalist doctors to specialist doctors. As the baby boomer (75 million people in the USA) generation ages, the need for generalist doctors to care for them is increasing faster than the supply. There are numerous proposals to solve this mismatch, but given that the United States has a strong cultural value of freedom of choice in choosing your profession and an aversion to any kind of "central planning" regarding such things there have been no great solutions. There have been proposed various incentives to entice doctors to the primary care practice of medicine including loan forgiveness programs, supplemented income programs, and the like but the trend has not really been changed. Simply increasing the number of medical school "seats" and training more doctors is not thought to be able to solve this mismatch either since it will likely lead to more specialists, but not be guaranteed to produce more generalist physicians. For now, the mismatch is being solved with the increasing use of "midlevel" providers—Physician Assistants (PA) and Advanced Practice Nurse Practitioners (APRN) to fill the unmet need for generalists. But that trend is also failing since the specialists have found the utility of PA's and APRN's in their practices as well and are attracting many of these midlevel providers to work for them in the specialty fields. These factors taken together explain why there are so many foreign born doctors practicing in the United States.

Also, the "match" just starts the post graduate training process for medical students. Technically the match just gets them an internship slot—the first year after graduation from medical school. To continue on the new doctor needs to subsequently get a position as a "resident" physician in the desired training program such as Internal medicine, surgery, Family Practice, OB/GYN, pediatrics, etc. These "residency" programs usually range from 2 to 3 years' duration after the completion of the internship year. Many of these areas have "subspecialty" areas as well—cardiology being a subspecialty of Internal Medicine for example—and so the resident physician who wants to get a "specialty" in those areas will need to apply for a training slot in a program that trains that type of doctor. It is up to the individual physician to arrange for his own slot in the desired training program. In the end, the new doctor will spend a minimum of 3 years, and as much as 7 or more years' post-graduation from medical school before launching into their career as a physician.

Another aspect of this process is the payment for post graduate medical training. Hospitals that have interns and residents in training programs obviously incur extra costs for their training. Interns and residents are paid stipends and are not charged tuition, and the program directors and other physicians who participate in the training of these doctors are also compensated for the time they spend teaching and training the fledgling MDs. In the past these costs were compensated by an increase in payment to the hospitals for medical care given to patients with an adjustment to the usual Medicare reimbursement received by the hospital. This continues to be the case. However, in this age of climbing medical expenses and in view of the efforts being made to curtail the increase in Medicare costs CMS (Center for Medicare and Medicaid Services) is not planning to expand these extra payment amounts to hospitals. The problem this causes should be obvious: as we increase the number of medical students trained and graduated there needs to be a concomitant increase in the number of post graduate training slots. But, with no increase (and actually talk of decreasing the level of payment from CMS) in payment from CMS to support graduate medical education we could be faced with an increasing pool of medical graduates but a stagnant or decreasing pool of post graduate training opportunities. This is a currently a hotly debated topic by policy makers. It could either result in no increase in post graduate training seats which would not increase the number of doctors trained which doesn't answer the need for more medical doctors as noted above. It may also reduce the opportunities of foreign trained doctors to come to the United States for training thus increasing the proportion of native educated practicing doctors (assuming we have an increasing pool of interested native born students). Or it may result in the imposition of some central planning and regulation process regarding graduate medical training perhaps taking away a part of the free choice of medical students as to what area of medical practice they may want to pursue for their careers. Another option might involve making the medical graduate pay for the cost of their post graduate training thus increasing significantly the accumulated debt required to enter the practice of medicine which would in turn reduce the motivation of young college students to enter in to the profession of medicine in the first place (and especially into those areas of medical practice that take 5 or more years' post-graduation to qualify the practitioner). Asking patients to bare the extra cost if they seek medical care at a teaching hospital is against the American way especially since a majority of hospital costs are paid by either Medicare or Medicaid. Many of the poorest members of our society receive their hospital care at teaching hospitals and public hospitals and they have no money to pay for even this basic care, let alone paying a premium to be cared for in a teaching institution. Is the payment for the education and training of medical doctors a responsibility of the public—aka the government, or should the cost of making new doctors be borne by the students themselves? This feeds into the major social policy question of our current generation: Should the United States continue the provision of medical care (both hospital and clinic care) in the setting of privately owned and operated hospitals, clinics and health care practitioners, or should the US go to a government owned and operated health care system? Stay tuned! The answer to that question will likely be decided within the term of the next presidential administration.

Internship and Residency

First a little education about the terminology of this phase of becoming a doctor. This time is generically referred to as "post graduate medical education" in which the medical school graduate—already an "MD"—gets the actual hands on training in the science, art and technology of medicine. In order to qualify for a license to practice medicine a new doctor must pass through a year of "internship" and then pass the part B test of the National Board of Medical Examiners. So after 4 years of medical school, plus one internship year, plus successful passage of the NBME part A and B exam, the new doctor is qualified in most states to practice medicine and could decide to "hang out his shingle" as they used to say and start to see and treat private patients. Doctors who do this are usually referred to as "general practitioners". In the past (4 to 5 decades ago) this was a fairly large percentage of physicians, but in this age of increasing complexity and technology in medical care very few do so now. A "general practitioner" defined as above is really not qualified to be a competent medical practitioner. So, most doctors pass through their internship and then continue on into a "residency" program that gives them a minimum of 2 additional years (and often more) in their specialty. At the end of that "residency" period they may then advertise themselves as a qualified medical practitioner in that field and start their clinical careers. Most residency programs lead to a certification examination in the area of specialty. So, for example, an aspiring pediatrician completes medical school and receives their "MD" degree, then serves their internship year followed by an additional 2 years of residency experience. (Other specialties may have up to 6-7 additional years after the internship!) Only then are they qualified to practice pediatrics. Most will also take and pass the pediatrics certifying exam given by the American Board of Pediatrics at which point they become a "board certified" specialist in pediatrics. If that pediatrician, then wants to become a pediatric cardiologist they must complete additional years (usually 2 or more) in a pediatric "fellowship" training program and pass another exam given by a specialty board. Only then can they advertise themselves as a "board certified pediatric cardiologist". If you are shopping for a doctor, you want to choose one who is a "board certified specialist". This designation can give you the assurance that you are seeing a physician who has taken the time to learn their area of medicine well enough to be a competent doctor.

Another piece of general information is needed to understand this phase of post graduate medical education. Interns and residents are often referred to as "house officers" in the training hospitals. They are in most cases technically employees of the hospital and are paid a monthly stipend or salary, have their malpractice needs paid by the hospital, and in the case of interns who are not yet licensed doctors practice under the supervision of the license of the hospital. A decade or so ago, these house officers were the only hospital based doctors but now in the last 10-15 years hospitals are also staffed by physicians known as "hospitalists" who are fully trained and licensed doctors. These doctors are also employed by the hospital but are not in a training program but are working as fully trained doctors in the care of patients in the hospital. This often causes confusion among the patients. Some hospitalists are part of the training staff for the interns and residents, and some are not depending upon the way the individual hospital organizes it. So when a patient is admitted to the hospital they may be admitted to the "teaching service" in which case they are cared for by interns and residents who are supervised by the post graduate training medical staff doctors, or they may be admitted to the "hospitalist service" in which case there are no interns or residents involved in their care. Either way, the patient is not usually seen by their out-patient doctor unless he is a specialist who admitted them for a specialty related illness. In our modern time most office based doctors who are not surgeons turn the care of their patients who need to be in the hospital over to the "hospitalists". This is often true also for the specialist doctors who may admit a patient to the hospital for a specialized procedure or care but will involve the hospitalists or the house officers to provide all the non-specialized care. This situation is compounded when the hospital also trains "fellows" who are fully trained and certified doctors who are in training to become specialists (such as cardiologists, neurosurgeons, etc. They may be a fully trained and certified internal medicine specialist, but be a cardiologist in training.) If you are confused by this imagine being an 80-year-old sick person who is also unnerved about whatever illness has brought them to the hospital! That patient will see more doctors than they can keep track of and will often be confused about who really is in charge of their care. Add to this the possibility that a medical student may also be assigned to the patient's care, and that some of the specialist doctors may have an NP or a PA working with them also see the patient and you have now completely befuddled the poor patient and their family. But there does not seem to be any other way to organize it and allow for the supervised teaching of new doctors to bring them to the level of experienced and competent practitioners of the art and science of medicine and surgery.

    Medical school runs on the usual academic calendar with the school year running from fall through winter and ending in the spring. So most medical students graduate in May and are ready to start their internships in June. They have been seasoned a bit as medical students, but this is the first time that they are truly on the front line of patient care in the hospital. My first day as an intern involved a brief orientation to the hospital—for me I had spent time in the LDS Hospital as a medical student so I knew where everything was. We were given several admonitions to "first do no harm", then given our assignments to different parts of the hospital and to the resident who we would be working with. Then we were required to pass certification in CPR since we would be first responders to patients in the hospital who might suffer a cardiopulmonary arrest—a "code Blue". Then off to the hospital "wards" to start our internship in earnest. Usually the house officer "team" consisted of two interns, supervised by one resident and with ultimate supervision by one of the hospital teaching staff doctors. Depending on the hospital service there may also be one or two medical students on the team. This represents a pretty green and inexperienced team to be taking care of sick hospital patients and there is a wide spread feeling that for the months of June through maybe September patients are at some hazard being taken care of by this group of doctors in training. There are layers of supervision by experienced doctors, but the interns and residents are the first layer, and are often the first to see the patient upon their arrival in the hospital and the chances for diagnostic and treatment error is fairly high. Wisdom comes from the proper application of knowledge and these new house officers are full of knowledge, but not yet full of wisdom!

So you start your internship. Now is the time that a newly minted MD starts to feel like a real doctor! You are called "doctor" and even though some unknowing patients called you by that title while you were a medical student, this time you know it is true. You are proud and feel great when you can introduce yourself as "Doctor Anderson" to your patients. You even get more respect from the nurses, physical therapists, and other hospital coworkers. You even get paid! When I started my internship in 1977 my salary was $10,000 for the year! I had never made that much money in any single year up to that time. It felt like I and my family were on the way to "Easy Street". In today's world, the average intern earns between $40,000 to $50,000 for their year. The rate of "pay" increases a few thousand dollars per year with each post graduate training year so that the new doctor can afford to live without having to borrow money. That is a good thing since the average doctor is already $100,000 or more in debt when they finish medical school. Most student debt contracts have to start to be repaid starting one year after graduation so the "big bucks" that they are making in their internship year soon start to face the realities of paying for the medical education. But this is the time that the 20-year-old clunker you have been driving may be able to be replaced with a 10-year-old "new car". A few of my cronies even purchased small homes during their post graduate years. In my case we moved out of a high density student apartment complex to a single family older home on the lower Avenues of Salt Lake City. (We weren't sure if it was originally a home or a converted chicken coop but it was "home sweet home" for us for the three years of our post graduate training.) But even though we were not making big money we did not feel poor and the prospects for our financial and social life were definitely looking up!

The internship year is demanding. Just the work hours would be daunting to any normal person. An intern's day starts at about 7am and continues for about 12 hours. Usually first on the agenda is making "rounds": this involves seeing the patients that are already in the hospital that the intern is caring for. They need to be assessed for any new testing needed to establish a diagnosis, or to see how they are responding to the prescribed— "ordered"—treatments. The intern usually writes these orders and is overseen by the resident and the attending doctor. Next comes team rounds were the interns plus the resident and medical students plus the attending doctor see the patients as a group. Here often the intern gets grilled about their assessment and their orders for treatment. This is meant to be educational but is often very intimidating and the intern does not want to be found lacking in the appropriate response to questions. Some of the attending staff doctors are pretty tough and demanding and feel that it is part of their job to put the intern on the spot. The supposed point of all of that is to train the new doctor to think quickly and on their feet. The intern doesn't want to be upstaged by the other intern on the team and for sure not by the medical student! Each patient is seen as a learning lab for the intern so the patient's particular problems lead to focused reading and studying by the intern in whatever "spare" time they can find. Then after rounds the day of work starts…sometimes it starts even before rounds are done.

    The intern functions as part of a team usually consisting of two interns, one resident and various medical students. There are commonly 3 such teams at the same time on any hospital service so the patients in the hospital are cared for by different teams. They may have different attending doctors or the same depending upon the training program's organizational plan. One of these teams each day is designated as the "on call" team and they are the admitting team for that day. Patients admitted to that hospital service are then admitted by the on call team—usually the two interns alternate taking admissions. Admissions may come from the emergency room or from private physicians' offices. In a typical busy teaching hospital each intern may admit 4-5 and up to 10 or more patients. The admission process involves patient assessment, writing orders for diagnostic testing and treatment. Each patient could easily take an hour to admit and unfortunately multiple admissions may come simultaneously so it can be a busy and hectic challenge to deal with. The resident also sees these patients but in a more abbreviated manner to be sure the intern has done his work appropriately. The on call team works all of one day, including overnight, and through the next day—so 36 hours—before being able to go home and rest and rejuvenate. The next day is a usual 12-hour day, and then back on call again. In my time it was not unusual for the intern to physically be in the hospital 100 to 110 hours a week. When you do the math and see that a week has only 168 hours in it and most of us mortal humans need about 8 hours of sleep (56 hours per week) there is very little time left over for anything else. An intern has no social life, very little family life, and no time at all for recreation. (During the first 3 months of my internship I only attended church with my wife and family a few times leading the members of our church to think that my wife was a poor young widow with 3 small children!) And, depending on the situation the night "on call" may not, and usually did not allow for much sleep at all since the interns on call not only admitted night time patients but responded to new urgent problems of patients for the other 2 teams that were not on call that night. The theory behind all of this time in the hospital is that the intern needs to get as much experience as possible with a variety of patient problems, and to do that you have to be there when they—the patients-- show up! Emergencies by definition are not scheduled, and the rare medical problem shows up rarely, so "if you snooze you lose!"

All interns are sleep deprived and most residents are as well. In fact, the whole experience of medical school and post graduate medical training leads to a sleep debt larger than the monetary debt that the medical student incurred! That is why the medical profession runs on caffeine—coffee, Coke, Pepsi, whatever—and carbs (not the kind of diet any doctor would advise their patients to follow). When all the post-graduate training is completed and the doctor is finally able to start his medical career, there comes some respite in the schedule, but still most doctors report working on average 55-60 hours per week for the whole of their careers. If the intern is married, it is a substantial stress on the marriage and divorce rates are high among physicians in training, and among doctors as a general group. If the young doctor has any non-medical interests, they have to be put on hiatus until some future time. No time for golf, heck no time for anything but a shower, a meal and some sleep at home, then back to work. No time to pursue romantic pursuits. No quality time with family or friends. Doctors are often described as "workaholics" and the term is aptly applied. And worse than that, they want to be busy and busy-ness is a badge of honor for doctors. If you see a group of doctors conversing, you can bet on it that at least one of the questions they have asked each other is "are you busy?" and no doctor wants to answer that in the negative. This "busy-ness" habit translates into offices full of patients waiting for doctors who seem forever behind schedule and too rushed to spend the time that the patient wants, or even needs, attending to the patient's complaints. Add to that the cost of running a medical practice and the decreasing level of reimbursement for patient care that physicians are experiencing in this decade and you have a recipe for sleep deprived and stressed doctors and patients who are less than satisfied with the physician-patient encounter. All of these factors have led to what is known as "burn out" that many physicians are feeling in this generation which leads to: doctors who appear to be uninterested in the patient as a person; who find no satisfaction in the practice of medicine; who focus more on "money" and less on patient care; who exhibit problems being empathetic to anyone including their families; who are ill-tempered and easily upset; who are more prone to making mistakes; who are depressed and prone to alcohol and substance abuse; and this is resulting in a trend for more and more physicians to quit medical practice in their 50's rather than continuing practice for a full career—thus aggravating the already mentioned problem of a shortage of physicians in the United States. There is a lot of conversation going on presently on how to help doctors deal with "burn out" but for now it is conversation only with no apparent solution.

    In the last decade there has been a pull back from requiring physicians in training to spend so many hours in the hospital. The current guideline now is to limit the hours the intern and resident spends "at work" to 80 hours! Proponents of this point to the higher probability of medical errors made by sleep deprived and stressed young doctors. Certainly there is something to that argument. But the old school pattern of 100 hours plus in the hospital is making a resurgence in the last few years because there is a very real thinking that the young doctors training experience is lessened by not being there in the hospital to take care of the medical experience they need to have. It is also suspected that many of the young doctors falsely report their hours at 80/week but are spending more time than that so they don't miss interesting and educational clinical experiences. There has even been a study recently that purported to show that surgical errors where not more common in surgical training when the doctor worked 100+ hours as compared to only 80 hours. There is even some talk of lengthening the internship and residency programs a year or more to make up for what is missed by restricting the work hours to 80 per week. Those doctors of my vintage think that this newer generation of doctors are all "wimps" -- since we survived the 100 plus hour schedule they need to buck up and do it too! The new generation of doctors all think we old grey beards are nuts. It may be that all doctors as a group are nuts. Surely the rigors of getting a medical education, the length of time and the greatness of the cost are major reasons why there is a decreasing interest among US college students in a career in the medical profession. A recent survey (Medscape Young Physician Compensation Report 2016) reported that only 60% of physicians under age 40, and 53% of physicians over age 40 would choose a medical career if they had to do it over again! That is a reflection of the total stress picture of becoming and being a doctor.

Right now you are all in the mood to read about my particular experiences as an intern. Well, that was 40 years ago and my memory is not so good as to be able to remember the individual stories accurately. It was an exciting and challenging time and I was young enough to survive the rigors of the schedule. What was interesting to me would not likely be interesting to you, and besides, doctors develop as a side effect of their education and experience a rather unique view of the world of sickness. If you have ever sat as a non-physician among a set of doctors who are casually talking—like at a social party, dinner, etc.—you will likely be grossed out and maybe even offended by what doctors think is amusing and conversation worthy! As a group what doctors think is funny does not fit the usual description of humor among the polite lay population. And detailed descriptions that involve blood and guts and other body fluids, or delirious or demented patients, or exciting medical misadventures are often unpleasant conversation for the normal person. If you want to read an interesting and all to true account of what it is like to be an intern I would refer you to the novel *The House of God* by Samuel Shem—I know you can still get it on Amazon.com.

The basic principle of internship and residency training can be expressed in the statement: "see one, do one, teach one." This applies to procedures like starting IVs, placing subclavian catheters or bladder catheters, doing CPR, performing a surgical procedure, etc. as well as to evaluating a patient in the ER with chest pain, or fever, or a seizure, whatever. This is why it is important to be at the hospital so much because you don't know when the next opportunity to "see", or "do" or "teach" may come along. Usually the resident gets first choice, the intern second and the medical student last. This then has doctors who have first seen the procedure progress to doing the procedure and finally to teaching the procedure. You can get only so much information from a textbook and then you need some hands-on experience. Going repeatedly through the process of "see, do, teach" is how doctors become competent practitioners. It is true that until you can "teach" the technique or procedure you are not really competent in its application. The conversation in the house officer's lounge among the doctors in training is almost totally about "interesting cases" that have seen, done or taught. By this means a wealth of experience is built up. As a house officer you hope to be able to "see, do or teach" every possible illness or procedure. Surgical residents keep an actual log of how many of a particular surgical procedure they have been involved with since certification as a general surgeon involves a certain minimum amount of experiences. Most hospital training programs have "Grand Rounds" which is usually a noon time group conference where interesting and unusual cases are presented and discussed. Also, all hospitals have "Mortality and Morbidity" (M&M) conferences where patients who die or suffer significant complications of treatment are discussed. These are all learning experiences for the intern and resident. The ultimate M&M experience is an autopsy of a deceased patient and although this is much less commonly done than in years past it is a very revealing process to witness and to learn from. This along with continued textbook study helps to round out the education and experience of the fledgling doctor.

There is an aspect of post graduate training that is often referred to as "town vs. gown". Essentially all hospitals that offer post graduate training are large hospitals with a full complement of physicians representing all specialty areas of medicine. But given that, there is a division: the hospitals which are associated with medical schools all have attending doctors who have academic appointments at the medical school and hold academic rank such as professor, assistant professor, associate professor, etc.; the other hospitals are staffed by doctors who practice without academic rank in hospitals that are not affiliated with medical schools. There is competition and even some antipathy between these two groups. The "gowns" are the academic doctors who often see themselves as the most competent authorities in their geographical area in their fields. These doctors are often involved in research and are often focused on publication of their research in the many medical journals. They teach medical students and physicians in training. They may be super specialized limiting their practice and research to a very narrow spectrum of medical or surgical problems. In times past they only took patients on referral from community based physicians—the "towns"—and by nature of that often looked down upon their community based colleagues as somehow less qualified or knowledgeable. Also these academic based doctors did not practice full time and often split their time between patient care and medical research and in fact they progressed from associate professor to professor based upon their academic pursuits and publications and not upon their ability to actually provide medical care to patients. The community based physicians are often more experienced in actual patient care because they do not split their time between patient care and other activities. They are no less qualified than the "gowns" but often feel they are made to look "second class" by the academic doctors. They often feel that the "gowns" are out of touch with the realities of medical practice and are insulated from the real issues of patient care by virtue of working in the "ivory tower" of academia. This problem is magnified by the fact that government agencies often look to the "gown" physicians for advice in formulating public policy (government regulations and payment issues, etc.) and the more experienced patient care givers—the "towns" are left out of the picture. It is the "gowns" who get interviews on the news, testify before congress, get invited to sit on advisory panels, participate in formulating policy, and are quoted in the newspapers. Thus the community based physician is left having their practice interfered with by government and insurance company policies that did not allow for their input in the decision making process. If the aspiring post graduate doctor wanted to become an academic physician (a professor of medicine or surgery) they needed to do their post graduate work at a university hospital among the "gowns" since there is very little crossing of the "gown" vs "town" line except in the direction from "gown" to "town". The distinction between "town" and "gown" has become blurred in the last few decades as public funding has diminished for the support of academic doctors who mostly did research and thus had their income mostly supported by government research grants and did not do much actual patient care. Most medical schools nowadays out of financial necessity (they need to fund their programs from revenue derived from actual patient care and not just from government grants and tax derived sources) have expanded to employing physicians of the "town" variety to staff outpatient clinics under the banner of the academic institution, but these physicians do not have academic rank other than "adjunct" professor which basically designates a physician who works for an academic medical organization but in a non-academic role. If you think that by going to a Medical University Health Clinic you are going to be cared for by doctors who are "professors" of medicine and surgery and thus will be taken care of by the "best" doctors, then you are mistaken. That is not to say that these doctors are not qualified, only that they are not in the "gown" group of physicians. All of this leads to my bias that if you want to be cared for by the most qualified and experienced physician you need to seek out the best community based doctor (a "town") rather than going to the most prominent university based "gown" physician. This rule may be modified in the case of very rare or unusual illnesses or for medical procedures that are highly specialized which tend to gravitate to the super specialized "gown" doctors who have a special research interest in these unusual problems. The academic doctor may possibly "know more" about a particular medical or surgical topic in which he is doing active medical research but the community doctor has clearly done more actual patient care and every medical study on the topic has shown that the best medical and surgical outcomes come from the care provided by the most experienced (in terms of actual number of patients treated) physician. Of course, you would expect me to have this bias since I did my post graduate training at a "town" hospital—and I practiced as a "town" doctor-- but I found that the community hospital training exposed me to a broader and deeper variety of actual patient care than I would have been exposed to in the "gown" environment (I did my medical school clinical work in a "gown" environment so I know of what I speak).

Once the post graduate physician has completed their internship and has passed the Part B National Board of Medical Examiner's examination they are eligible to apply for a license to practice medicine. This application involves presenting your credentials to the State Department of Professional Licensing (DOPL), and paying a fee and a license to practice "medicine and surgery" is granted. In addition to a State license, another license is needed to be able to prescribe medications. This license comes from the State and Federal Drug Enforcement Administration (DEA). These licenses are State specific so if you want to practice in a particular State you must get licensed in that State. Additionally, if you want to be able to admit patients to a particular hospital you must apply to that hospital for admitting "privileges" and you will not be allowed to admit patients or give medical orders for any patients in the hospital unless you have those privileges. The process of gaining hospital privileges involves submitting an application with proof of DOPL and DEA licenses as well as letters of reference from physicians who have observed you practice and can attest to your competence. Many, but not all post graduate physicians apply for and get licensed by the DOPL and DEA at the end of their internship year, although that is not required to continue in the post graduate training program. In decades past it was common for doctors to finish their post graduate training after their internship and start their private practice as "general practitioners", but that is a rare thing nowadays and I would be very wary about going to a doctor with that minimal set of credentials. But, getting licensed after your internship allows for the opportunity to "moonlight" which is a way to earn some extra income while getting some additional medical experience albeit non supervised.

Moonlighting is a common practice. It provides two things: extra income, and extra experience. The income is nice because most loan programs for medical school ask for repayment to start one year after graduation. Some moonlighting income helps to keep your cash flow up and avoid needing to borrow more money. The extra experience is nice, but it comes with a lack of close supervision so there is a bit more of an opportunity for some medical misadventures! I moonlighted at two venues. The first was flying in a medical helicopter or airplane ("Life Flight") for medical transfers to the hospital where I was a house officer. After I had completed my intensive care unit rotation and passed that with a good recommendation I was qualified for flying "life flight". I was the physician present for transport. We usually were pretty well informed about the patient and the medical problems before leaving to pick up the patient, but often the patient was more sick than advertised or in small outlying hospitals and was not well diagnosed so there was room for surprises. Occasionally we would get to the referring hospital and a different patient than we went for was felt to be higher priority so that we ended up picking up something we had not prepared for in advance. The most memorable patient for me was a trauma patient that had come to the ER of a small hospital while we were enroute and was not the patient I thought I was going to get. Upon arrival the patient had a pneumothorax—a collapsed lung-- and needed to have a chest tube placed. I was the doctor that needed to do that...problem was I was in the "see one" phase of chest tube placement but had never actually put a chest tube in a patient. But reminding myself silently that "the complications of a chest tube are managed by a chest tube" I got the job done without showing too much uncertainty to those who witnessed and was able to get the tube in properly and stabilize the patient for transport. It was cool and adventurous to fly medical transport but after a highly reported crash of a medical helicopter in the Midwest with all on board being killed in the crash my wife convinced me that my career as a medical "cowboy" was over! Having at the time 3 children with a 4th on the way I conceded her point. But, nothing was cooler than "saddling up" in the Life Flight helicopter and heading for some small rural hospital to pick up a patient. The other moonlighting, I did was as an ER physician in a small rural hospital in south-central Utah. This was a busy ER being near the interstate and the only hospital within a hundred miles in any direction. I usually worked a 24 or 27-hour shift on the weekend when I was off duty at my house officer job. I saw a little bit of everything in that ER including auto trauma, gunshots, knife wounds, industrial accidents (it was a coal mining town), fevers in young children, heart attacks, strokes, pneumonia and sundry infections, drug overdoses, and even delivered a few babies. I interpreted my own x-rays since the radiologist didn't come in until Monday morning and I was always worried that I might miss a cervical fracture in head and neck trauma patients. In that small town, on the weekend it seemed that all of the community physicians became very scarce and I was essentially the only doctor within a 100-mile radius! I admitted some patients to the small community hospital for the community doctors to see on Mondays. I usually saw 60 or more patients during my shift and got very little or no sleep. I worked about 2 shifts a month for nearly 2 years and I don't know how I didn't die during those two years from sleep deprivation. I had a 120-mile drive home after my shift was over usually getting home about 11 pm Sunday night and needing to be at the hospital Monday morning at 7 a.m. Like I said earlier in this monograph, the medical profession runs on caffeine and I usually had a full tank of the stuff while I was in the ER. What I couldn't handle I tried to stabilize and then sent on to the bigger hospitals up north by ground or air ambulance. I learned quickly to depend upon the very experienced nursing staff that worked beside me and often just asked them what they thought I should do. I don't remember a time when they steered me wrong. My rate of pay for both of these moonlighting jobs was $20/hour which in 1978 and 1979 seemed like I was robbing the bank! But in retrospect, I am sure that the doctor who I worked for in the ER easily collected $1000 or more for my services and paid me $480 was the real bank robber in the situation. Nowadays, no ER doctor would consider working for less than $150/hour. But hey, the extra income was great and the experience was more than I could have gotten in any 24-hour shift as a house officer.

    Outpatient clinic was part of the post-graduate program, but a minor part. I had a 4-hour clinic once a week and in that 4 hours saw maybe 10 patients on a busy day. I had 30 minutes or more to spend with each patient and I was not rushed. I didn't have to deal with phone calls, requests for medication refills, calls from the emergency room, drug reps, "emergency" appointments, or any of the stuff the usual doctor deals with many times a day in their clinic schedule. My total patient cohort could not have been more than 100 patients. I really don't know where these people came from. I suppose they got clinic care at no or low cost and they knew that I was a physician in training. I had a few of the usual types of medical problems including high blood pressure, diabetes, chronic heart disease and arthritis. One of the hospital teaching staff was there with me so I could ask for help with anything I needed. One advantage to those patients was that I had all the time in the world to spend with them. Of course, this experience was to teach me a little about outpatient medicine but it did not do the job. This clinic experience was nothing like what clinic practice is like in real life. In real life clinic practice for me was 25-30 patients per day in 15 minute intervals with a lot of distraction along the way from patient phone calls, requests for prescription refills, questions about insurance and billing issues, multiple drug salesmen wanting just a few minutes of my time to talk up their latest "new drugs", telephone calls from the hospital about patients I had there or from the Emergency Room about patients of mine that had landed there or worse unattached patients that I didn't know for whom I was the "on call" internist. Clinic practice occupied 10+ hours of my day every day when I got into my private practice. The post-graduate training in out-patient medicine was the least fun, and the least fulfilling of the "see on, do one, teach one" regimen of post graduate training. There was absolutely no training about the non-medical side of running a clinic. Nothing about scheduling, billing, collections, strategies for handling phone calls, paper work, insurance government red tape including pre-authorizations and pharmacy formulary restrictions. We had little exposure to handling patient complaints, family issues, or other aspects of the "art" of medicine. The clinic staff were employed by the hospital so human resource issues were not on our training palate. At least in the time that I was in training (1977-1980) the internal medicine doctor was well tutored in the care of patients who were sick enough to be in the hospital, but poorly tutored in clinic patient care. When I got into private practice I was comfortable with the care of sick hospital patients, but taking care of ambulatory patients in the clinic put me on a very steep learning curve. I had to learn how to treat ambulatory patients without any mentoring other than from my clinic partners. This is one reason why so many internal medicine graduates now days opt to go into "hospitalist" practice rather than clinic practice and is a reason why there is such a shortage of "primary care" internal medicine physicians in the United States. Clinic practice is demanding, exhausting, frustrating, intense, and pays poorly compared to hospital practice. The current added demands of government and insurance companies, the continued suggestion that primary care doctors screen their patients for everything from domestic abuse to whether or not there is a gun in the house, the increasing interference of regulations with drug prescribing, preauthorization for tests and procedures, and the continuously changing landscape of documentation and coding and billing and other insurance "red tape" is the reason why primary care doctors are suffering from "burn out" at an alarming rate of over 50%! In recent polls of office based doctors well over 50% of those who are 50+ years old admitted that they are thinking of quitting. Doctors who practice in the outpatient clinic setting are overworked, under paid and worse are under appreciated. In recent years internal medicine trained doctors tend to go first into hospitalist practice (50-60%), or on to subspecialty practice (20-25%) and last into outpatient clinic practice (15-20%). Internal medicine trained doctors are currently very high on the recruitment list of companies that recruit physicians to available practice openings. This trend has increased over the last decade with no sign that this issue will change in the near future. This is the major reason why NPs and PAs are becoming the most common primary medical care providers in our nation. The NPs and PAs are now asking for licensing that allows them to practice independent of MDs and would allow them to set up their own medical clinic offices without any affiliation with MDs. Studies have even been done to attempt to show that NPs and PAs provide outpatient primary care that is equivalent in quality to that delivered by MDs. (These studies have looked at a very few diagnoses such as hypertension and diabetes which have highly defined guidelines for patient care. Most NPs or PAs are not good at evaluation of a patient who comes in with non-defined symptoms.) This trend is just starting and is sure to increase to the point that at some time in the next decade MDs will be in the minority as primary medical care providers. In fact, most physicians who specialize in Family Practice or office based Internal medicine are now referred to not as doctors but as "health care providers" a term that seems equally applied to PAs and NPs. The consuming public will soon think of NPs and PAs as equivalent to MDs. Primary care physicians are now the Rodney Dangerfields of the medical profession who complain that "I don't get no respect!" They are not happy being designated as health care "providers" instead of MDs! NP training programs that used to graduate NPs with a masters-equivalent degree are now transitioning to PhD-equivalent degrees and NPs will soon be known as "doctor". With the nation-wide shortage of MDs especially in primary care these NPs and PAs are fast filling up the medical offices that provide outpatient care to our citizens. Even in specialty clinics such as cardiology or gastroenterology the doctors employ NPs and PAs and these are the practitioners that the patient most often sees first when they go to these specialists rather than the doctor. It used to bother me immensely when I would refer a patient of mine to a cardiologist or a gastroenterologist or some other specialist only to have them seen by a PA or NP instead of the doctor! I felt then and still do that I was more qualified than the PA/NP and what I really wanted was an opinion from the specialist MD! Time will tell if this trend benefits or degrades the medical care outcomes of our citizens but with the coming physician shortage this is how the future looks. Good news for PAs and NPs—jobs are abundant.

    So the time came in June, 1980 when I had my medical license, had completed all the required time and experiences to qualify as a board certified internal medicine specialist (I had to take a written test in September of that year and pass it before I got the "paper" stipulating that I was board certified) and was ready to go out into the world and practice medicine. I paused for just a moment to consider going on into one of the subspecialties (I considered pulmonary medicine and gastroenterology) but decided that since I was 30 years old, had four children and $25,000 in debt (this was 1980) it was time to start to make my place in the world. So, look out world here comes Dr. Anderson!

Hanging out your shingle

Decades ago it was common for a physician starting their practice to open an office and start to try to build a patient clientele. It was not uncommon to see small physician groups ranging from one to 5 physicians. All that was needed was a suite of offices/exam rooms, a receptionist/secretary/nurse and some basic equipment like exam tables, BP cuffs, and maybe some basic office surgical equipment for suturing, splinting and casting, etc. Some specialties were more equipment intensive, especially ophthalmology, but the basic office set up was not too expensive. Essentially no education was given to the doctor in training about how to do any of this, nor was any given for the basic business skills involved in billing and collections, insurance issues including claims coding and submission, liability issues involved in running an office, employee benefits and management, government regulations regarding medical practice and a host of things that are part of running the business part of medicine. The new doctor just fumbled their way through this all, learning as they went. Their first employee was often their spouse who served as scheduler, secretary and receptionist. That was a gentler and simpler age! Nowadays the business side of medical practice is so complex and specialized that the new doctor needs to have employees who are trained and experienced in all of these issues. (An article in the Harvard Business Review September 23, 2013 was informative of this trend: from 1990 to 2012 health care jobs increased 75% with 95% of this growth represented by non-MDs; the ratio of doctors to non-doctors was reported as 1/16 with 60% of the non-doctors in purely administrative, non-clinical jobs. This 1/16 ratio represents a cost per doctor for non-MD personnel of $823,000. No wonder health care costs in the US are going out of sight!) Whereas in the past a doctor may need one or two employees to run their business, now the average doctor needs 5 or 6 employees. Employees or consultants to advise in compliance issues of the government and insurance companies are essential and add to the non-MD ranks of health care workers. The overhead cost of running a medical practice usually is 55-60% of revenue. So if the doctor wants to have a personal income of say $230,000 (this is roughly the average yearly income for primary care physicians) they need to generate $550,000 in collected revenue to do so! If the physician wants to start saving for retirement they need even more collected revenue to do so. And remember payment for educational debt starts one year after graduation from medical school. The first years of a medical practice can be fairly lean for the new physician as they build a patient clientele, establish an office, start to pay back student loans, look to purchase a home for their family, and maybe update their 15-year-old car for a newer model. If their business is slow to grow they often look for places where they can augment their income like moonlighting in the local ER or working in nursing homes. Most primary care physicians who venture out starting their own practice have many lean income years before they really start to take home the income they thought that they would make. But the average physician in the "good old days" had an independent spirit and was desirous of being in control of their medical career. All of these issues were just an exhilarating part of being a "real doctor" at last. But because of these many factors most new physicians today look to start their practice in an established medical practice that has all of the necessary infrastructure in place and offers them a guaranteed base salary. These factors are the main reason why the days of the 1-5 physician medical clinic are over and gone! And nowadays 88% of primary care doctors and 85% of specialty doctors start out their practice as employed physicians often working for a hospital or a large insurance company. (Data from Medscape Young Physicians Compensation Report 2016.) This saves them from the cost of establishing their clinic and staffing it as well as from the need to get up to speed in the business part of medical practice management. They just show up with their stethoscope and that is it! I started with an established physician owned and operated medical clinic group being the 7th doctor to be part of that group. I had a guaranteed first year base salary of $35,000 (1980 dollars) with all the infrastructure already in place and functioning. I became a full partner sharing equally in the overhead expense after the first year. Eventually over the next 35 years our medical group grew to over 150 physicians by absorbing many smaller physician groups under our business umbrella. The advantages of being a large physician group include some "economies of scale" that help to lower overhead a bit, and the ability to offer on-site medical services such as X-ray, lab, physical therapy, outpatient technical services (that would otherwise need to be done at a hospital) that can augment income and improve patient care and satisfaction. This physician-as-entrepreneur era however has nearly come to its end. What few independent physicians and small physician groups are left are rapidly selling their practices to become employed physicians working for some big health care company or hospital. The days of small and large physician owned and operated medical clinics are fast disappearing in the rear-view mirror of history. Hospitals and medical insurance companies are now the owners of most outpatient medical groups. Nowadays most physicians who finish their training look for an employment situation with a big medical group that provides all of the infrastructure for them and offers a guaranteed salary from day one. No need to take out a small business loan to start up a medical practice using your wife as secretary/receptionist/accountant/manager and sometimes nurse, just show up with your stethoscope and go to work! And unfortunately, with medical practices now being just a part of a bigger impersonal health care company the personal service that patients may remember from the "doctor down the street" is gone, never to return. And it is not only the patient that loses but the physician becomes just one of countless "health care providers" managed by some big bureaucratic organization.

    In the past, it was the minority of physicians who were "employees"—who were hired by and worked for some business entity that was not physician owned or operated. Most academic doctors were salaried employees of a University Medical School. Some private clinics also developed where the doctors were salaried employees such as the Mayo Clinic, Cleveland Clinic, etc. But the majority of physicians were not employees, but worked as individual entrepreneurs either singly or in small groups. They were physician owned and managed. Nowadays the opposite is the rule. Most physicians look for and are hired by some private business entity and work as employees of that organization. The major employers are University Health Care systems that hire many physicians to staff their outpatient practice venues, big insurance companies who own hospitals and clinics and hire physicians to staff their clinics, and some large private business entities that employ physicians such as the Kaiser Permante Health Care system.

Only in rural areas and some inner-city ghettos do you still find physician owned, small group clinics. The trend in our day is for "vertically integrated" health care systems that own and operate medical insurance companies, hospitals, clinics, home health care services, ancillary health care services and physician services. Physicians then are just a part of the big business entity and are subject to having their salaries, schedules and benefits dictated by non-physician managers thus losing the freedom of self-management that was such an attraction to doctors of old! The trend of the last few decades is such that if we don't soon end up with a nationalized health care system with doctors as federal government employees, we will end up with maybe 5 or 6 mega-health care businesses that run extremely large vertically integrated health care systems and control all of health care services between them. Doctors are already being debased and devalued in such systems being labeled as "providers" rather than "doctors/physicians" and are considered in the same way any business considers its other employees. The satisfaction of physicians with their medical practices is falling significantly as this trend grows. The major complaints of employed physicians is that their clinical lives are controlled by some non-medical MBA-trained manager whose only consideration is the financial "bottom line" for their business. "Bean counters" dictate medical care and physicians must follow the company imposed rules and regulations. Physicians feel undervalued, depersonalized, and controlled by people who have no idea about how to provide medical care to actual patients. They don't feel that management listens to their legitimate medical care concerns regarding their patients. Management imposed schedules, quotas, production targets, along with controlling the hiring and management of physician support staff has left many physicians sufficiently dissatisfied with medical practice as to look for early retirement or non-clinical jobs. Patients complain that physicians are robotic, distant, unengaged emotionally with them, rushed, abrupt, and don't take time to listen to their concerns. This is all due to the fact that the traditional physician-patient relationship that supports all of those positive things that patients value is seriously degraded in the physician-as-employee business model. Add to this the fact that current Medicare rules and programs are forcing physicians to forge unnatural alliances with diverse physician groups—such as "Accountable Care Organization" (ACO) groups and we have in my opinion a recipe for a crisis in physician provided health care on the near horizon. Although small, there is a growing call among physicians to form physician unions to allow for the power to negotiate with the management side of these health care behemoths. In the nationalized health care systems of western Europe physicians are already represented by unions and several "strikes" have taken place to force management to negotiate with the physicians. Is this the future of health care in America?

Another modern trend of medical practice has been termed "doc in a box". In this arrangement physicians who offer primary care services are employed to staff small walk in clinics. These are often termed "urgent care" clinics, but physicians may be found in small venues like shopping malls, large airports, or other nontraditional practice locations. Even big box stores like Walmart are considering having these services in their stores ("WalMed"?) The motivation for this is to capture the patient who has a sudden health complaint for a quick, non-comprehensive, and often impersonal health care encounter. These venues are often staffed by physicians who have not been successful at building their own private clinic practice, or who do not have any desire for a long-term physician-patient relationship, or who are moonlighting to supplement their income as they start up their clinical practice, or who are physicians in training looking for extra income. Often these sites are staffed by PAs or NPs with some supervising arrangement with a physician who may or may not be on site in real time. These physicians are often transient, and are not looking for a long-term practice venue to spend their career in. They are all salaried and managed by whatever business entity owns the "box" they work in. Patient satisfaction is generally not high with this arrangement other than for the convenience factor. The main advantage is the walk in, no appointment needed availability of the patient seeking medical care. The patient does not expect to establish a long-term physician relationship and the doctor doesn't look to establish a long-term patient clientele.

A disturbing trend from a physician's point of view has come into play with the emergence of advanced practice nursing professionals—so called "nurse practitioners" (NP). Initially NPs were seen as "physician extenders" who could help the physician they worked for care for their patients. Especially now when primary care physicians are in short supply and the number of older patients is increasing as the baby boomers enter their golden years, NPs and PAs (physician's assistants) have offered a way to extend the physician's ability to care for more patients. At first NPs were licensed only to work under the association with a supervising physician. However, in recent years in many states licensing for NPs has allowed them to work independently from physicians essentially acting not as physician extenders but as physicians. In years past NPs had a master's degree level of training, but now many NP programs are producing PhD level training and degrees for NPs. As a result of this NPs have been pushing to be allowed to have clinical practices independent of physicians and without physician supervision. A recent controversy was set off as the Veteran's Administration has decided to grant NPs hospital privileges in VA facilities without requiring physician supervision. This is setting up the boundaries of a "turf" war between M.D.s and NPs that is just getting starting but will surely result in the decision to allow NPs to have fully physician independent practices in the coming years. Especially in the primary care arena, it is entirely predictable that as the next decade matures more and more primary care practices will be served by NPs and not MDs. PAs have not yet started to push for independence from physicians but count on seeing that also in the coming years. Studies are already being published that promote the assertion that the medical care provided by NPs is equivalent to that provided by MDs. Just at a time when the nation needs to be making it more attractive rather than less attractive for MDs to go into the primary care fields, NPs are pushing their way into that area of medical care. It could easily be predicted that at some future time all primary care providers will be NPs and only specialists are MDs. Of course, from the perspective of a national health care agenda NPs offer an obvious advantage over MDs since the currently accepted/average salary range for NPs is in the range of $105,000 compared to MDs in primary care averaging maybe twice that amount. But don't expect NPs to be satisfied with the lower salary and they will undoubtedly push for payment parity with physicians. It is not inconceivable that once NPs have saturated the primary care practice market they will look to start to establish themselves as qualified specialists as well. The crisis in primary care medicine will have some interesting solutions in the future!

And, now a new trend is developing that has long been thought to be a poor venue for a medical encounter: Telemedicine. In this type of medical practice, a physician is connected to the patient over a secured internet connection with video capabilities. Of course, the medical interaction involves a very limited repertoire of services mostly relegated to verbally consultative care. But just in the last few years the trend is increasing and insurance companies are now starting to agree to pay for some of the services. This virtual "doc in a box" may expand to become a part of physician services that augments the services offered through an established medical clinic to established medical patients, or it may develop into its own patient-physician care entity that is independent of any physician's clinical office. A variation of this is also emerging where a robotic "doctor" consisting of a video monitor, attached to some equipment such as vital signs measuring equipment and access to some patient data including labs and x-ray reports with mobile capabilities that can move from patient to patient who may be in a hospital or a nursing home allowing physicians at a remote location (? home in their pajamas) to have virtual interaction with patients. Maybe this new patient care module should be called "doc in his pajamas"! A higher tech version of this currently exists even for doing surgery where a robotic machine is at the patient's side in the operating room actually doing the cutting and sewing all the while being controlled over the internet by a doctor who is not even in the same zip code. "Virtual" medical practice may become a viable practice venue for the coming generation of doctors. In the areas of chronic disease management this "virtual doctor's visit" will likely provide financial economy and will become more and more attractive to insurance companies who pay for the services. If equivalence of outcomes can be shown with virtual doctor's visits compared to in-the-office visits then expect this to be an exploding trend in the future.

Another option for hanging out your shingle for the physician is hospital care. In the past, a private physician would see his patients both in the clinic and in the hospital. That was great for the hospitalized patient who would be taken care of by a doctor that "knew" them. However, for the doctor it was not so great because hospitalized patients often required his attention at inconvenient times during clinic office hours, weekends and evenings. Hospital patients represent a

24/7 commitment for the physician. In physician group practices this was handled by having physicians in rotation being "on call "for the hospital so that all of the doctors in a particular group did not have to be on call for hospital patients every night and every weekend. But over the last 3 decades and especially the last 10 years this issue has been addressed by having full time hospital physicians—so called "hospitalists". These physicians do not work in the clinic but only in the hospital. They admit, take care of and discharge the patients who are sick enough to need to be in the hospital leaving the clinic physician free of the burden of taking care of patients in both locations. This practice has matured enough now that almost in any hospital of any size, even in rural settings, the hospitalized patients are taken care of by "hospitalists". These hospital doctors are well trained and expert in taking care of the sick hospital patient. But there is a downside to this as well. First, the hospitalists as a group are very transient and often work at any particular hospital for only a few years before seeking employment in some other location. And second, once the patient is well enough to go home their care is transferred back to the clinic doctor. Unfortunately, the clinic doctor may not have been aware that the patient had been in the hospital and thus uninformed of the details of the illness, what was done, any medication changes, and any needs for timely follow up. The potential exists for the baton to be dropped as it were in the transition from hospital back to clinic in such a way as the patient ends up being readmitted to the hospital because of inadequate or untimely follow up. Medicare now has identified a hand full of hospital diagnoses and follows those patients to see if readmission to the hospital for the same diagnosis occurs within 30 days. If so the hospital is fined by Medicare—fined by having a reduced Medicare reimbursement rate for all hospitalized patients. This is an issue of significant import and there are multiple ideas being floated about how to address it. Some solutions are entirely unacceptable to the clinic doctor such as having "post-acute" clinics staffed by the hospitalists to follow up with patient after hospital discharge. This would further remove the office based physician who does most of the care of these patients from being involved in the follow up of these people. All sorts of solutions are currently under consideration to improve the "handoff" from the hospitalist to the clinic doctor. It is fair to say that the problem is not yet solved. Also, there are some potential conflicts of interest between the hospitalist and the clinic doctor since essentially all hospitalists are employees of the hospital and subject to their manager's rules and regulations, but many of the clinic doctors are not employed by the same entity, or may be independent practitioners. There is room to fight over "whose patient is this!" between the two groups of physicians. The problem is aggravated by Medicare ACO organizations that hold the reimbursement of clinic doctors accountable to pay for the cost of hospitalist services. This is not a happy arrangement. It is providing motivation to vertically integrate all physician provided care under a single pay arrangement such as a nationalized health care system or a vertically integrated private insurance company management. Time will tell how this works out, but in my estimation the hospitalist trend is another factor that will eventually lead to a nationalized health care system. The hospitalist practice of medicine is continuing to evolve. There are now in some hospitals physicians who only do OB care/deliveries, or who do only pediatrics, or who only provide night coverage for specialty doctors (these doctors are known as "nocturnalists"). There are even a few hospitalists who are dermatologists and only take care of skin issues in hospitalized patients! It may soon come that in the USA there will be a full complement of hospital physicians of all specialties who practice exclusively in the hospital, and a similar full spectrum of clinic specialists who only practice in the outpatient venue. This arrangement is already the rule in many European nationalized health care programs. This trend stands to likely increase hospital costs for patients since the "general hospitalists" will be apt to consult the "specialist hospitalists" more and more often thus multiplying the number of doctors involved with the patient and increasing medical charges. Coordinated medical care of the patient may suffer from too many physicians each taking care of only a single body part of the patient. The culinary wisdom that "too many cooks spoil the porridge" applies when there are multiple specialty doctors who take care of the patient but none who assume the overall management. Thus hospital costs increase, the patient ends up with too many doctors and medical care becomes less efficient and more cumbersome and fragmented, and the clinic practicing physician is left out of the loop thus compromising their ability to adequately take care of the patient once they are out of the hospital.

Finding Patients and building your practice

Back in the day the newly minted doctor hung out his shingle, advertised his willingness to see new patients and then waited for them to come to him. The process of building a practice involved a welcoming attitude and availability. Associating with an established doctor always helped so long as there was an unmet need for more physicians in the community. Hospital emergency rooms often referred patients to the new doctors in town and word of mouth referrals from satisfied patients built the practice. But nowadays those simple techniques won't do, and they don't work. Most private insurances are organized around "Preferred Provider Organizations" (PPO), or "Health Maintenance Organizations" (HMO) and in order to be able to serve patients insured under those arrangements the new doctor has to be accepted as a "provider" in the insurance network. This is no easy job anymore since many such networks are closed to all but employed physicians. Some networks decide administratively how many of what specialties of physicians they need to service their enrolled patients and limit the number of doctors allowed on the panels to a specified number. You as the new doctor in town may not be able to get onto those panels and have access to those patients. Even Medicare has HMO plans that restrict their patients to certain health provider networks and if you are not one of those physicians you are out of luck! Medicaid also has preferred provider networks. Self-pay patients are always looking for a willing provider but in many cases self-pay means no pay for the doctor. Patients insured under standard Medicare or Medicaid are free to choose any willing provider but many physicians quickly find out that if their practices are full of standard Medicare or Medicaid patients their income from their practice may just only cover their overhead expenses leaving them practicing for nothing! Physician's often belong to State or County medical associations and also often belong to national organizations of physicians in a particular specialty and these organizations are active in trying to promote "any willing provider" access to insured patients, but in the end it is the insurance companies that have the power because they have the money. This problem can be very daunting and because of this many newly minted physicians seek employment with some medical service company that already has a captured supply of patients (by means of medical insurance enrollment) to "feed" the new physician's practice. These practice arrangements come with non-MD administrators and all of the disadvantages to the physician that were noted in the above comments about "hanging out your shingle." In recent years there has been a rebellion by some physicians (with increasing numbers opting for this choice) to establish what has been termed "concierge" practice or "direct primary care" practice. In this arrangement, the primary care physician offers essentially unlimited office visits including office lab tests to their patients in exchange for a set enrollment fee paid by the patient directly to the doctor. Typically, the enrollment fee may be from $1,500 per year to $50-75 per month per patient. For that fee the patient gets all primary care services at no extra charge, or in some arrangements a small "copay" at the time of service. The patient pays the fee, and the service is available. In this scenario the physician needs to have about 500 patients to generate $750,000 in collected income per year. This makes this option attractive but it is still in its infancy in the United States. The physician does not deal with the insurance company (if the patient has insurance) and hospital services are not included. This type of practice arrangement is being talked about among physicians so much that you cannot read a magazine that deals with medical practice that doesn't have an article or two about this. Whether or not this practice arrangement will flourish depends upon whether or not the US moves to a nationalized health insurance plan in the next few years. If it does not expect to see these new types of medical practice increase in number across the country as doctors shed themselves of the administrative burdens and red tape of dealing with insurance companies. A nationalized health insurance plan ("Medicare for all" it is often termed) is a highly likely probability in the next presidential administration if there is a Democrat in the White House, and then all bets are off about what the private practice of medicine will look like. Physicians may become public service employees, or more likely will be private contractors who have to deal with only one payer source—the government—under whatever rules and regulations are promulgated. In that scenario all private medical insurance goes away and the government controls everything. Then "provider panels" and other restrictions regarding physician participation will be gone and replaced with some new and possibly equally onerous regulations. If physicians do not become federal employees under a nationalized health care plan then expect to see physicians form labor unions for collective bargaining with the government. And, if there is a national health care plan with physicians as employees or as private contractors you can also expect to see a steep rise in the number of "direct" primary care physician practices, but since their patients would have to pay out of pocket for care they otherwise could get for "free" (you know—government funded "free"!) there will be only a small minority of citizens who would participate in this option—most likely the financially well-off who can afford the luxury of paying for more personalized medical care than they would get from the "Medicare for all" plan.

    The times we are in now leave the newly minted physician with uncertainty about how their clinical practice career will turn out. The majority of newly minted doctors are choosing to be employed physicians working for the government or some large healthcare company, typically an insurance company. It is only a distinct minority of physicians who go into practice as "their own boss". Times past a career in medicine attracted the independent personality who desired to own and manage their own practice and either singly or in company with a physician owned and operated clinic chart their own rules and regulations and be in charge of their own practice arrangements. Studies are now being done trying to contrast these two groups of physicians (independent physicians vs. employed physicians) in terms of income, hours worked, satisfaction with their practice, satisfaction with their management type, and personal satisfaction with the practice of medicine. Most of these studies suggest that either arrangement is roughly equal but each with different advantages and disadvantages for the physician. Given that, I think the times favor that most if not all new doctors in the next decade will be employed physicians in medical groups managed by non-MD business managers. The few who do not will be in some kind of "direct primary care" arrangement as described above. The patient will be the loser in all of this since the physician will respond first to whoever pays their salary following all the rules and regulations from their employer, and will have the patient's preferences and needs as a secondary consideration. For me, I am glad I am now retired since I had personal issues even with the physician management of the group I was a part of for 35 years. I railed against insurance companies and government regulations so much that the thought of being employed by either of those entities makes me cringe.

Getting paid

A little bit of history is in order for this topic. Before about 1960 medical insurance was uncommon and Medicare and Medicaid were not in force. Patients got sick and when they exhausted their home remedies went to the doctor who treated them and charged them a fee for the service. This "fee for service" arrangement had some drawbacks for both the patient and the physician. For the patient the fee had to be paid from their personal financial resources. Most physicians adapted their fees to be affordable for their patients. There was no standardized fee for a particular service, and the patient could negotiate with the physician about the fee and its payment. Some fees were paid "in kind" with a barter type arrangement. Physicians commonly billed on a "sliding scale" fee schedule based upon their patient's ability to pay. Patients often avoided seeking medical care because of the expense and then would present with illnesses that were quite advanced and harder to successfully treat. But then, medicine was not as advanced then as now and many illnesses did not have established and proven therapies. The concept of preventive health care services was not yet the standard of care and screening tests and preventive health care services were minimal. On the other hand, the physicians were respected members of their communities but were not necessarily wealthy (unless they inherited their wealth) making a better than average income but nothing compared to today. The "patient-physician" relationship was direct and personal and intimate. There were no insurance company or government mandated intermediaries between the patient and the physician. Perhaps those days were a gentler and kinder era?

Then in 1965 (two years before I graduated from high school) the Medicare and Medicaid legislation was passed to provide medical insurance for those over age 65 and for younger persons with disabilities and for those who were on public assistance payments. Private medical insurance through some employer groups began to be more common as well. Since then both Medicare/Medicaid and private health insurance has expanded to its present behemoth size and US health care spending (public plus private) now accounts for an amount equal to 17.5% of the nation's GDP or $3 trillion dollars in 2014 which represents $9,523 per person per year! Obamacare (the Affordable Care Act of President Obama) has further expanded the insurance coverage of the American citizenry, but still leaves about 20 million Americans uninsured. Healthcare spending is now the largest Federal expenditure accounting for $1.4 trillion dollars in 2016 making it 22% of all government spending! Healthcare is now big business and if you look up just about any medium sized city today on Wikipedia and look at the list of the largest employers Healthcare employers commonly rank first or second (they usually vie with public education for first place). This has had many effects upon both patients and physicians. Now, most American citizens (90%) have some type of medical insurance. They have preventive services available and coverage for physician office services and for hospitalization. They no longer have to worry about whether or not they can afford to go to see the doctor or go to the hospital. Physicians have seen their incomes increase as the US has matured from a patient to physician fee for service arrangement to a medical insurance to physician payment arrangement. Physicians now are among the wealthiest of the citizen population. Careers in health care—both as practitioners as well as administrators—have become among the best paying occupations. But the patient physician relationship has become strained and insurance regulations and red tape have been interposed between the patient and the physician. Physician fees are set by the insurance companies. Patients are required to pay "copays" for medical services that are not negotiable. Patient access to the physician of their choice is restricted by HMO and PPO arrangements. Medical services are available but need "preauthorization" by the insurance company. Patients and physicians have both become in effect commodities to be managed by those who pay for health care…i.e. "managed health care." Health care "miracle cures" abound and the ability of diseases to be effectively treated has expanded exponentially, but the delivery of medical care has become subject to business models and business management. Medicine is "big business" in the biggest sense!

When I started practice in 1980 I joined an internal medicine group of 6 physicians in Provo, Utah. By then Medicare, Medicaid and private insurance coverage had matured a great deal and in large part physicians and hospitals provided services, sent the bill to the insurance companies and were paid what they billed. Looking back these years between 1980 and 1990 may have been the "golden years" of medical practice in the United States. Patients had better access to medical services and physicians were starting to get paid much more than in the preceding era. Physicians as a group started to enjoy a "boom" time in regards to their income and physicians joined the ranks of the wealthiest in their communities. This resulted in health care cost inflation, and for the citizens who lacked health care insurance coverage medical care became even less affordable than before. There was a minimum of regulations and red tape for the physician to deal with, and there were no restrictions about what patients the physician could provide medical care for—no HMOs or PPOs, etc.

I remember in the early and mid-1980s our group of 7 physicians regularly had 60-70 patients in the hospital at any one time. Many were there for "tests" that are now routinely done as outpatients. Many were there for treatments that are now done out of the hospital. There was no length of stay guidelines or rules for hospitalized patients. As a group of MDs we had to have 2 of us "on call" on the weekend so that we could see all the hospitalized patients and also respond to the Emergency Room and new hospital admissions. But most of these patients were not really very sick by today's standards for hospital patients. Soon Medicare and private insurance companies started to realize that the that they were spending a lot of money! So, Medicare came up with the solution known as "Diagnostic Related Group" (DRG) payment for hospitalized patients. Basically, Medicare established a payment amount for the hospital care of a patient with a specific diagnosis—for illustration let's say Medicare would pay $5000 for hospital services to treat a patient with pneumonia. This DRG payment was all that the hospital would get, but they would get that amount whether that patient stayed in hospital 2 days or 20 days. It didn't take long for hospital administrators to see that they had to cut the length of stay of patients or they would go bankrupt. Suddenly there were put in place all kinds of prospective and retrospective reviews and regulations that severely restricted what patients could be admitted to the hospital and how long they could stay. Hospitals put severe pressures on their physician staffs to comply and within a year of this system being put in place our 7-member physician group went from having 60-70 patients in the hospital at any one time to having 15-20 patients in hospital! The patients in the hospital were sick, were there for treatments that needed to be done in the hospital, and as soon as they recovered sufficiently to be able to manage at home were discharged. Hospital administrators changed from strictly facility managers to patient managers. Physician autonomy was curtailed by rules and regulations.

At the same time as the DRG system for hospital payment was put in place, the system for payment of physicians was modified. No longer would the physician submit a bill and be paid the specified amount. The insurance carrier would decide what amount to pay the physician based upon the description of the service or procedure. There had been in place for over 50 years a statistical classification system of disease known as the International Statistical Classification of Disease (ICD) sponsored by the World Health Organization as a way of classifying diseases for the purpose of statistical analysis. This system gave a numerical code to a diagnosis—Hypertension for example was "401", diabetes was "250". However, with the advent of insurance payment for medical services the ICD codes were adopted to numerically classify diseases and treatments for the purpose of determining payment amount and then came many rapidly applied revisions and expansions so that the current iteration of ICD is ICD-10. The Medicare DRGs utilized the ICD system and hospital payments were tied to particular ICD codes. In ICD-10 now the codes have been expanded to 3 or 4 digits after the main code—so Hypertension may now be 401.111 (illustration only) to describe hypertension with some particular set of sub-characteristics. It is now required for the hospital and for the physician to correctly "code" the ICD number for a given patient so as to be able to submit a bill for payment. The imperative to apply the correct code—and to apply the code that allows for the highest amount of payment—has led to a whole new medical profession: medical coding. All hospitals and physicians must have employees who are expert at coding the bills with the proper ICD codes in order to maximize billing to the insurance payer. Additionally, a separate code (known as Current Procedural Terminology—CPT—codes) was developed to represent numerically what the physician did—what service or procedure they provided—and that code is used to determine what specific monetary value will be provided for payment for that service. These codes have specified standards that must be met to justify one level of payment as compared to another. So, to submit a physician bill to insurance the physician needs to specify the correct ICD code and the correct CPT code for the service they provided to the patient. This has all led to the imperative of electronic billing with specified ICD diagnostic and procedure codes…all resulting in the multiplication of businesses that provide the computer software to do this properly. So no longer does the patient see the physician and the physician provides a service for which payment is received from the patient—no, now the patient sees the doctor from a list of insurance approved physicians on their "panel", the physician provides a medical service, the physician's office (or hospital) crafts a bill with an ICD code and a CPT code which is digitally sent to the insurance company, the insurance company examines the codes and tries to find a way to down code them to the lowest possible reimbursement amount, and then the insurance company pays the physician. The overhead cost to the physician or hospital is substantial under the current arrangement and may be as much as 25% or more of the reimbursed amount for the cost of computers, coders, accounts receivables clerks and business management personnel. When you factor in the cost of property for medical office/hospital, utilities, licenses, management, etc. the overall overhead for medical services easily reaches 55-60% of collected revenues. No wonder the healthcare industry in the USA constitutes so much of the GDP.

   Back in the "olden days" physicians charged a fee that they determined by themselves was a fair price for their services and modified this fee often on a sliding scale based upon their perception of their patient's ability to pay. Some physicians would even provide free care to selected patients. This allowed the doctor to cover their expenses, make an acceptable income, and to adjust their fees to the circumstances of the patients they served. All this changed when insurance became involved. Medicare started out paying fees based upon a "usual and customary" pay scale that more or less represented what the average fee for a particular service was from a cross section sampling of physician bills submitted. Subsequently in 1989 a system was devised called the Resource-Based Relative Value Scale (RBRVS) for physician payment that took into consideration the physician's work for a particular procedure or service, their practice expenses, and their malpractice expenses. This formula then was used to compute a "relative value" number for the physician's service. Practice work expense variables include the relative cost to the physician of becoming qualified to provide the particular service—it costs more to become a neurosurgeon than and family practitioner for instance. Practice expenses for providing a service are higher with some physician specialties due to office equipment required such as an ophthalmologist who need multiple expensive devices to provide their services. And, malpractice costs vary widely among specialties—for instance in many locals the malpractice expense to be an obstetrician may be as much as $100,000 per year compared to a family practitioner who does not do obstetrics paying maybe $5,000 per year. All of these variables were considered and then a Relative Value Unit (RVU) was computed. Finally, that RVU was multiplied by a number representing a geographic area of the USA on the presumption that the costs of practicing medicine in some area are more than in others, and a final RVU was established for the physician's service. So, a RVU was established for each CPT coded service and payment then was determined by that calculation.   In this system "procedures"—i.e. things that physicians might do to the patient such as surgery, biopsies, scope exams, radiological procedures, etc.—were more highly valued than "evaluation and management" services—services that the physician provides that are not procedural such as managing hypertension or diabetes or treating an infection and the like. This resulted in the broad variation of physician incomes that we see such that neurosurgeons and orthopedic surgeons are among the highest paid medical specialties and family practitioners and pediatricians being among the lowest paid specialties. All insurances including Medicare, Medicaid and private insurances adopted this system. Traditionally the physicians fee that was submitted for payment to the insurance company would often be much higher than what they got paid—as much as 200-300% higher because the insurance would pay only what the RVU formulation computed. That is why when you look at your explanation of benefits form from your insurance company you may see that the orthopedist charged $40,000 for your knee replacement but the insurance only paid them $8,500 as an example. This is true for hospital bills as well. In this system it doesn't matter what the physician charges as their fee, the payment is determined by the ICD and CPT codes and the RVU for that particular procedure or service. This payment arrangement rewards the physician for the quantity of services provided—if they do more they get paid more. The incentive to the physician in this system then is to do as many "units" of service or procedure as possible to maximize their income.

Over time Medicare costs increased as the factors of the RVU increased payment to the physicians. Rising practice expenses and malpractice costs as an example would increase the RVU value over time. Inflated costs of medical equipment and such also increased overhead costs to the physicians and was adjusted for in the RVU system. The costs also increased due to the fact that doctors increased the number of services provided in response to the incentive to do more and get paid more as well as for increasing demand for their services. Medicare developed a "sustainable growth rate" (SGR) formula that by law set a limit on how much the payment to physicians could grow yearly based upon the predicted increase in Medicare funds available to pay those fees. Predictably this SGR rate was significantly less than the inflation in physician expenses as calculated by the RVU formula, and the increasing number or services. The SGR rules stated that if the rate of increase in physician expenses exceeded the SGR rate, then the Medicare payment schedule would be reduced to keep Medicare expenses within the SGR guidelines. Every year then for decades as the Medicare fiscal year end approached dire predictions were made about how much the reduction in Medicare reimbursement to physicians would be. This of course led to an increasing uproar from physicians with threats to stop taking care of Medicare patients all together! Of course, this would not do so congress would always step in at the last moment and vote in a modification to the SGR rule to allow for no reduction, and usually a small increase, in Medicare payments to physicians. There was no end in sight for this yearly ritual until in 2015 Medicare changed the rules...MACRA (Medicare Access and CHIP Reauthorization Act of 2015) became the new reimbursement model for Medicare.

MACRA represents not just a new rule for physician payment, but a radical departure from the old way of paying out Medicare funds to physicians. The old SGR rule no longer applies but is being replaced by MACRA. It is coupled with two other acronyms—MIPS (Merit-Based Incentive Payment System) and APM (Alternative Payment Models (APM). These new rules are new and not (as of this writing) published, but they are in place to make a fundamental change in how Medicare pays physicians. Basically, the new system proports to pay physicians for "quality" and not "quantity" of services. It also intends to link physician payments to health outcomes as defined by Medicare. Its intention is to reward physicians financially if certain patient care metrics achieve preset standards, and to financially penalize physicians if they fall below the standards. The promise is that if physicians alter their practice patterns enough to ensure that they provide proper quality services to their patients they will be rewarded for the decrease in quantity of services with an increase in reimbursement. A requirement to be able to comply with MACRA, MIPS, and APM rules will be for the physician to be able to document in their electronic medical records (EMR's) that they have met the Medicare established guidelines for providing quality "outcomes" for the patients they take care of. Complying with these new rules will increase the physician's costs of providing patient care since the rules specify certain reporting requirements that will either take physicians away from patient care to comply with or more likely will require the physician to hire additional office staff to comply with. The legislation aims to be budget neutral so for any physician whose Medicare reimbursement increases due to total compliance another physician's reimbursement must decrease. Most physicians are not happy with this new arrangement! Many small medical practices (single or small groups of physicians) have pointed out that the increase costs to them for complying with these requirements will of necessity increase their overhead and reduce their income. Many physicians are presently threatening to withdraw from taking care of Medicare patients altogether because of these new rules. Physicians complain that "quality care" is not promoted, but that compliance with Medicare produced standards is what is increased. There is no current proof that Medicare standards actually make people healthier! "Quality" is a word that in this case means "compliance" and forced compliance at that with financial penalties for noncompliance. These new rules are a major motivator for physicians who are starting up nontraditional practices such as "direct primary care" as discussed above. I have often thought to myself and complained to my colleagues that if Medicare had set out with a stated goal to make complying with its rules so onerous that physicians would stop seeing Medicare patients, they couldn't have done a better job! And that was with the "old" Medicare before MACRA, etc. And that is not all! Part of the Obamacare legislation has mandated the formation of Accountable Care Organizations (ACO) in which physicians group together to form an ACO, then Medicare assigns a group of Medicare selected patients to that ACO. In that arrangement the ACO then becomes accountable for the total Medicare payments for that group of patients including hospital and ancillary care expenses! The ACO group may be rewarded financially if it can deliver less than expected expenses for the patients, and potentially penalized if that group of patients exceeds expected costs. (With so many diverse physicians in the ACO what this will result in is a "food fight" among medical providers each arguing with the other about blame for overspending and about who gets how much of the reimbursement.)

Medicare has another new idea for physician payment for hospital services that is bound to cause issues. In the past if a patient was admitted to the hospital and cared for by doctors who were not employees of the hospital Medicare would get a bill from the hospital and a bill from the physicians involved in the patient's care. So a patient admitted for surgery would have Medicare billed for the hospital and for each of the physicians who cared for them—the surgeon, the anesthesiologist, the intensive care doctor, etc., all separate bills. Now they are proposing moving to a "bundled" payment where a single global payment will be made by Medicare for that patient and this payment will have to be divided by the hospital and physicians for their shares of the payment given. The payment will be to the hospital and it will be up to the physicians involved to negotiate (i.e.

fight) for their share of the money. This will necessitate a discussion, negotiation and agreement among the hospital and the physicians about who gets how much of the money! Don't expect this interaction to be cordial since there will be much disagreement about the relative value of each party in providing the patient's care. The hospital will argue that since they provide the place and equipment for the patient that they should get the largest amount. The physician will argue that without them the patient would have not been in the hospital in the first place! Other physicians will argue that they provided relative more value to the care of the patient than the other guy. If the patient had complications, then the doctor who addressed the complications will argue that their service was the most valuable. This will lead to legal action, lawsuits, etc. as each party fights for what they think is their share of the compensation. The only way that this arrangement will work without serious fighting between the parties is if they are all "owned" by the same entity—hospital, doctors, etc. all owned and operated by some larger business be it private or government. In my opinion, that is precisely the point—to make all health care in the United States under the management and control of the government.

    Private insurance companies are not currently involved with MACRA type arrangements but experience teaches that ultimately what Medicare starts ends up being the model that private insurance follows. They however have for a long time used various other arrangements to try to reduce financial outlays for patient care including the now common HMOs, PPOs, and IPAs. They have even experimented in the past with plans that put physicians at financial risk if expenses exceed targets for patient care, and these plans are starting to resurface again after initial failures a few decades ago. These programs strive to reduce patient care expenses by requiring limited physician provider panels, limited hospital choices, limited drug formularies, preauthorization requirements for diagnostic tests such as MRIs and for surgeries and other expensive medical procedures. Private insurance companies are also involved in acquisitions and mergers so that it is predicted by some that in the next decade there will likely be only 4 or 5 large national private medical insurance carriers. Once they have that kind of control, expect more top down management decisions to dramatically affect physician practice and income. Private medical insurance is fast approaching a crossroads—if government insurance (Medicare and Medicaid) expands to become a National Health Care Service covering all US citizens then private insurance will go the way of the dinosaur. If, however, there continues into the next decade both private and government health insurance then the private sector will surely consolidate into just a few highly managed and tightly controlled business models. Either way, the physician loses…and if the physician loses the patient loses as well!

While on this topic of getting paid I need to talk a little about why many doctors won't see Medicaid patients, and even some will not see Medicare patients. It's all about money of course. Medicaid has the worst reimbursement schedule of any insurer. Given the fact that most medical offices have overhead costs of 55% or greater, the amount that Medicaid will pay for a physician visit does not even cover the doctor's overhead costs. I have often remarked that seeing a Medicaid patient is like giving the patient a $20-dollar bill as they exit the office and saying "have a great day and come again soon!" It is clearly a losing proposition. The only possible way to make any money seeing Medicaid patients is to run a "mill" seeing 50 or 60 patients a day at 5 minute intervals, and then it has to be in a bare bones practice setting with no medical amenities like on site blood draws, any ancillary testing, etc. and be primarily staffed by PAs and NPs. On top of that Medicaid patients tend to be among the most demanding patients coming as they do from the welfare rolls and used to government entitlements. They are well known as a patient group for missing appointments, failing to fill prescriptions, failure to comply with treatment recommendations and are frequent flyers at the local emergency rooms of hospitals. Then add to that the fact that the Medicaid red tape is without peer in being the most difficult to deal with. I always felt that I had a civic duty to see Medicaid patients but I kept them to not more than a few percentage of my patients—I would only accept one new Medicaid patient per month into my practice. Many doctors just refuse to see them altogether. That is why the "Medicaid expansion" part of ObamaCare will never work because you may end up with more patients insured by Medicaid but you will not find any greater number of willing providers to service their needs.

Medicaid also has a HMO product administered by Molina and you would have to be a fiscal idiot to participate with that organization as a physician. Medicare is only marginally better. Medicare only pays 80% of the "approved amount" of the physician's fee leaving the doctor to collect the 20% that the patient is responsible for. That 20% needs to be paid in cash by the patient or by a Medicare supplement insurance. Usually the pay schedule for office visits with Medicare is just marginally higher than your overhead costs per patient...if the 20% the patient owes is not collected then the doctor just covers their expenses but makes no profit for themselves. For doctors who do procedural stuff (surgery, scopes and the like) on Medicare patients the situation is a little better since most of that care is done at a hospital or surgical center where the facility absorbs the overhead cost and the physicians just have to pay for coding and billing and collecting services to cover their overhead. Many primary care physicians tell their patients who are retiring from their employment and thus loosing employer provided insurance and transitioning to Medicare that they will need to find another doctor to take care of them. I saw several new patients in my office each week that were in that situation. There is a story told about two brothers that decided to go into the water melon business. They bought water melons from the farmer for $1 apiece and trucked them to the city and sold them for $1 apiece. After a while they looked at their books and one brother remarked that they weren't making any money in their business. (Of course if you factor in their costs of doing business they were losing money on the deal!) The other brother remarked "yeah, maybe we need to get a bigger truck!" Medicaid, and to a lesser extent Medicare is much like the water melon business. The government feels that increasing the number of patients insured will do wonders for doctors as they will now have many more patients to fill their appointment books. But having a "bigger truck" does not solve the problem the doctor has of coving their overhead expense and having a profit left over with which to pay themselves for the work done and the liability accepted. We must ask the question: will a national health care plan do any better than that especially in view of the significant increase in costs assumed by the government to insure every single one of the 350 million Americans? The only way that can work is to make drastic cuts in the number of services offered—rationing by que—and to mandate very sharp pay cuts to physicians, hospitals, pharmaceutical companies and medical equipment companies. This will be a very difficult transition indeed!

How much money do doctors make?

To start out I must make a qualifying statement: when it comes to reporting income doctors as a group will understate what they earn! No, I am not saying that they underreport their income to the IRS, just that if you were to ask them how much they make you will get a "lowball" answer. I suppose this may be because they are embarrassed to be earning what they do, or maybe they are trying to be modest. Only when talking privately among themselves will the report of income approach the truth and that is only if they are talking to other doctors of the same specialty. (I once about 1985 overheard a fairly new plastic surgeon in our town complaining to a more established plastic surgeon that it looked like it might be 4-5 years in practice before he was able to make "a million" per year!) Another statement can be made that is also true: when asked whether or not they are being paid what they are worth almost all doctors will report "NO", and sometimes "Hell, No!"—just ask any primary care doctor. (A point of data that supports this is a recent review of orthopedist surgeons who are traditionally the highest earning doctors—over half reported that they were not satisfied with the amount of their income and thought they should be earning more!) And a third statement is true: most doctors when asked how many hours they work per week will overstate the amount of time that they actually spend in patient care activities. Maybe this is to make it look like the amount they earn is deserved because of how hard they work? I must say that the source of these comments is my own experience and observation and you will not be able to find much documentation in published reports that support these statements, but you can depend upon them as being true. That being said most doctors work about 40 to 50 hours a week and then when you add in the time that their time is really not their own because they are "on call" (even if they don't get called and have to go into the office or hospital), most doctors work week is 55 to 60 hours.

Doctors who are employed by some hospital or insurance company or large private clinic generally make a little less than their counterparts who practice privately. Women physicians as a rule make less than males, but it is unclear whether this is because they work less hours or because they are wage discriminated against as is the general case in other job settings. (ICD codes and CPT codes do not have a gender identified so if a male or female bills the same ICD and CPT code the reimbursement will be the same amount.) University professors of medicine or surgery often make less than their private practicing counterparts in salary, but the wage gap is often made up by stipends the professors get for being department chairperson, or on hospital or other corporate boards, or in research grant money, etc. Doctor's earnings are sufficiently high that some are able to work a part time schedule and still have a nice six figure income.

Doctors as a group clearly fall into the upper 10% of income compared to the general population and many of them are in the upper 1%. However, as most doctors will complain they don't make what rock stars, athletes or corporate CEO's make and that grates on them some---maybe not that they don't make those multimillion dollar salaries but because those who make those really big bucks didn't seem to have to put in all the time, effort and money to be able to produce that income compared to doctors. I suppose in that area doctors are not much different than the rest of the American public!

Some doctors will point out that it took a lot of time and money to be able to qualify to make what they earn. After all, it takes until age mid 30's and at a cost in educational debt of $200,000 to $300,000 to be able to even hang out their shingle and start to earn on their investment in time and money. Many doctors when they are grumpy will point out that the value their services add to the overall welfare of the population justifies such large earnings. (However, it could be argued that water and sewage department workers have contributed as much to the health and welfare of the American public as have doctors and they earn salaries that are 20% of what the lowest paid doctors earn! Do me a favor and don't ever throw that piece of information in the face of doctor that is complaining that they don't earn what they deserve.) When it is pointed out that in real inflation adjusted dollars the physician of today far out earns the physician who practiced in the days before Medicare and medical insurance you will not likely get a friendly response. Physicians have a love-hate relationship with Medicare and insurance companies, but it is absolutely clear that the financial life of physicians really hit its stride after Medicare and private insurance became the norm in the USA. (How many total hip replacements at a physician billed cost of $40,000 or more do you think an orthopedic surgeon would do if the patient didn't have insurance and had to pay the cost out of their own pocket? —I rest my case!)

Doctors who do procedures such as surgery, scopes, biopsies, heart catheterizations, etc. make on average 2-3 times what physicians who don't do procedures make. This is in part due to the inequality in payment that was part of the original RVU system that has been magnified as inflation has progressed. Because of this the "non-procedural" specialties such as pediatrics, family medicine, and internal medicine are the current most sought after doctors by physician recruiters because there is a shortage of these primary care doctors in the USA. It is no secret why this is. If we have a lot of orthopedic surgeons who practice 35 to 40 hours a week and not very many primary care physicians who practice 50-60 hours a week it should not take financial genius to understand why! There is a suspicion that more procedures are done in the USA than are really medically indicated based upon the presumption that more doctors are specializing in the procedural specialties and when you have doctors who are qualified to do a procedure more procedures get done. Now, in this statement I am really treading on sacred turf but there is at least a particle of truth in it. I was once told by an orthopedic surgeon when I was discussing physician incomes with him and complaining that us lowly internists don't make what we deserve that "Well, you could have been an orthopedist too if you wanted to earn what I earn!" When the doctor who does the procedure is also the doctor who is the one who recommends the procedure there is room for a conflict of interest. For now, I will let this topic rest on that statement.

So, how much do doctors make? Well, according to the most recent surveys the 4 highest paid specialties are orthopedic surgery, cardiology, gastroenterology, and dermatology. These 4 specialist groups average about $400,000 in income per year. (This is self-reported data from surveys. Remember my remarks at the first of this chapter. These amounts are seriously understated. A recent report by a doctor recruiting service reports that cardiologists are actively being signed to <u>starting</u> contracts for $525,000 and orthopedists to a similar amount with some contracts as high as $800,000!) Many of these specialists have financial interest in ambulatory surgery or endoscopy facilities and make additional income from the proceeds of those business entities. It is not unusual for these specialists to earn additional "passive" income up to $100,000 or more per year. Radiologists, neurosurgeons and other procedural specialties earn in the $300,000 plus per year range. Many physicians in these highly paid specialties make $700,000 or more per year! Primary care doctors such as family medicine, internal medicine, and pediatrics are at the bottom of physician earnings coming in at the $200,000 or less range. (It is interesting that the doctors on the lower end of the pay scale are more accurate in their self-reported incomes. The same doctor recruiting service noted above reports that primary care doctors are being offered first year contracts for about $225,000.) All the rest earn in the $200,000 to $300,000 range. So if the average orthopedist earns $400,000 per year and works 40 hours a week for 48 weeks a year they are paid $208 (more like $450 per hour if truth be known) dollars an hour for their efforts. A pediatrician who earns $200,000 per year and works 55 hours a week for 48 weeks a year earns $75 dollars an hour. These numbers represent net earnings and since medical overhead for physicians is in the range of 55% you need to double these numbers to get a feel for the gross revenue that physicians need to generate to achieve these incomes.

In the UK and Europe where national health care systems have been in place for some time physician earnings are substantially less than in the USA. Although it is hard to get your hands on good comparative data it appears that European physicians earn about one half of what their American counterparts earn. In the UK a general practitioner earns an equivalent of about $116,000 compared to a family practitioner in the US earning $220,000. An orthopedic surgeon in the UK or Canada earns an equivalent of $250,000 to $300,000 per year compared to the US orthopedist who earns $500,000 plus per year. What this translates to is a prediction that under a nationalized health care system in the USA all physicians in all specialties will have to take a significant pay cut. Don't expect that a single one of them will accept that without loud protestation. And expect that physician's unions which have heretofore had trouble getting going in the USA will become a rising political force in our future.

A Day in the Life….

So, what is it like being a doctor? First I will tell you what it is not. It is not glamorous like the doctors lives you see on the TV shows. No restaurant dinners every night. Golfing maybe but not every Wednesday. No instant wealth and privilege unless you are born with it. No invitations to mingle with the rich and famous. It is, like all other professions a job. It will consume your time and your energy leaving your "off" hours few and your energy depleted at the end of your day. It was once the case that there were two kinds of workers: the common man, and the professional man. The common man made his way in the world by his sweat and labor. The professional man had a life paved by the privileges of his rank and title. These are clearly long gone vestiges of a past time and place. True, some physicians feel that they have a "calling" to practice the art and science of medicine but their numbers are diminishingly small. More and more in our times the practice of medicine is only one of many vocational choices that can lead to financial satisfaction. It used to be that becoming a physician was the path to fame and fortune, but now with the high tech and business industries there are many other paths to the same financial and personal ends. It happens to be a vocation that is very time consuming and expensive to qualify for and because of that the number of young people who want to be doctors is decreasing. It is a profession that once you have finished your preparations to practice its art and science leaves you poorly equipped to seek any different type of employment if you become dissatisfied with the reality of the life style it requires. It is a profession loaded with 3rd party (3rd party being defined as anyone or anything that is interposed between the doctor and their patient) interference and in our modern times is not the vocation to choose if your personality doesn't do well with being tightly managed by endless rules and regulations that are developed and administered by people who know nothing of the art and science of medical practice. And finally, it is a vocation on the cusp of substantial changes in every way including science, technology, and the business aspects of medical care. It requires intelligence, commitment, hard work, adaptability, patience, forbearance and endurance. If that describes what you want for your life's work, then medicine is for you. If not, look elsewhere for your life's work.

Fortunately for those who choose medicine as a profession there is a very wide array of career choices. There are opportunities for research. There are academic possibilities for teaching. There are many clinical practice choices from the various medical and surgical specialties. The various medical and surgical specialties each provide a different experience with differences in lifestyle, income and practice. Unfortunately, given the length of time it takes to qualify to practice in one of the many specialty areas, if you should find after all that you really don't like the outcome of the choice you made there is no practical opportunity to go back, retrain and become something different. If you take until age 35 at the cost of $300,000 in educational debt to become an orthopedic surgeon and then find out after a few years that the practice or orthopedics is not really what you thought it would be, well, you are too old and too obligated to allow you to go back and retool as some other kind of doctor or to seek a non-medical career. There are some opportunities to do non patient care in administration, insurance consulting and some other jobs but they are few and are not likely to satisfy your long held professional paradigm.

I practiced as a primary care internal medicine specialist. That is the face of medical practice that I know. So the description of "a day in the life" that I will give is from that perspective. I don't really know what an orthopedic surgeon's day is like, or for that matter what a pathologist does all day so I can't really describe that for you. The first 28 years of my practice I had a clinic office where I saw patients and had privileges at 3 different hospitals to which I admitted patients, consulted on patients or took ER call. The last 8 years of my practice I worked as a hospitalist and did no clinic office practice.

My day usually started at about 5:30 a.m. when I would arise in time to get an hours' worth of exercise to try to keep myself healthy. My family consisted of a wife, and at full staff 8 children. Time to help my wife with breakfast, getting the children off to school, etc. then occupied me until about 7 or 7:15 a.m. Then off to the hospital or hospitals to make rounds on patients I was attending in the hospital. Most of the time my patients were in just one hospital, but at times I had patients to see in the morning at two different hospitals and that was very time challenging. Many days my "on call" partner had admitted a patient of mine to the hospital the night before so I was going in to see a patient whose problems I was only incompletely aware off. Normally I would have on average 5-6 patients in the hospital and it would usually take 2 hours to see them and direct their care for the day. Some days it would take more time than that and given the fact that they were sick enough to be in the hospital I had to attend to their needs first before going to the clinic to begin my day there. No time to chit chat with the hospital staff or other doctors about anything except direct patient care issues. Then off to the office which lucky for me was right across the street from the main hospital I attended at. Patient appointments usually started at 9 a.m. and hopefully I was done with the hospital work in time to be on time for the first appointment. My office day consisted of seeing 25-30 patients at 15 to 30 minute intervals. I never knew if the patients who had 15 minute appointments had a 15-minute agenda or a 30-minute agenda so staying on schedule was challenging. Hearing a patient say just as I thought I was done and was ready to leave the exam room "oh, by the way doc...." was all too common and it was a schedule killer. Most patients were understanding when I was running behind, but many weren't. But the truth was, my practice overhead was 55% and I didn't start to "pay myself" as it were till I was more than half way through my patient schedule. To see less patients per day was just not a viable financial option. Along the way through the day I had to keep patient charts updated, review lab and x-ray tests that had come to me from patients seen on previous days and decide if the results needed priority attention, respond to 40-60 patient telephone messages that detailed anything from a request for a prescription refill to a description of acute symptoms that needed attention, and negotiate a seeming army of drug company salesmen who all wanted "just a minute of my time" to hear about their drug of the day! (I finally decided that drug "reps" were to medicine what flies are to horses—you just can't get rid of them and you just have to ignore them the best you can.) On that topic, many physicians nowadays refuse to see drug reps because of the significant time interruption they represent. I usually took a sandwich to work for my lunch and ate it while multitasking all of the above issues. I drank a lot of Pepsi! Hopefully I was done seeing patients by 5:30 or so because I was usually left with about an hour of paper work to finish up at the end of the day. Any interruptions of that schedule by the hospital—either current patients who had taken a turn for the worse, a request from a surgeon for a consultation on one of their patients, or the ER wanting me to admit a patient to the hospital—blew my office schedule all to smithereens! These types of interruptions were common and occurred almost daily. Some hospital issues might require my attention at the end of the day, and finally with those things done I was home by 7:00 p.m. I was "on call" on average about once every 5th day and every 5th weekend and that involved taking new patient admissions from the ER, consulting on other physician's patients for medical problems as well as responding to patient care issues for my patients as well as my partner's patients in the hospital, with some phone calls from patients who were at home needing some medical issue attended to. I did take one half day (Wednesday afternoon) off a week which was necessary for me to be able to transact any kind of personal business in the community, or for other personal needs. I could not just leave the office at any time for even personal issues since that put me further behind schedule when I returned. My average work week was about 60 hours, and in addition to that when I was "on call" I was pretty much tied down because of a need to be available, even if I didn't get any calls. I often visualized my day as getting on to a treadmill with no opportunity to get off until the day was finished with me! This is the glamorous world of practicing primary care internal medicine.

    About 6 years before I left my office practice the hospitals I attended at hired "hospitalists" to take care of the hospital patients. I did not like this idea at the first since these "hospitalists" did not know my patients and my patients still expected me to be involved with their hospital care. My mindset was that I would take care of my own patients in the hospital so I had to learn a new paradigm. For a year or so that was a very uncomfortable strain, but finally I just had to let my patients know that if they ended up in the hospital some other doctors would take care of them and then when they were released from the hospital they would come back to see me in the office for follow up. There are still some "bugs" to be worked out with the hospitalist system because often I would see a patient in the office who had been in the hospital and I had no information about what they were admitted for, how they were treated, what medications might have been changed or what new medical problems had been diagnosed. Of course, the patients all thought that I was in the loop in real time and "had their records" but that was not the case. This is a problem nation-wide and it has not been adequately solved. Making it worse, new Medicare rules penalize financially the hospitals if patients end up being quickly re-admitted for a problem for which they were recently hospitalized so the hospitals have a motivation to make sure that doesn't happen. Some hospitals now are wanting to have their hospitalists (who are employed by the hospital) see recently discharged patients in an "after care" clinic at the hospital! Of course, that then puts the hospitals in direct competition with the office based doctors and it doesn't take a genius to see that the office based doctors are not happy with that in any way! Having hospitalists take care of your sick patients puts the primary care doctor in a love-hate relationship with the hospital. Being freed from having to make hospital rounds at the start of every day, and being freed from being "on call" at the hospital and the ER does free up some time for the office based doctor but it comes at a price. And now, Obamacare rules involving the formation of ACO's (see discussion above) put the primary care physician who is in the ACO at financial risk for what happens in the hospital—the most expensive venue for medical care-- even though they have no direct patient involvement there. This is an argument for a nationalized health care system (or a highly organized "vertically integrated" private insurance system such as the Kaiser system) that would allow integration of hospital and outpatient services which could then allow for a solution to these stresses on the physician.

    After 28 years of practice as I described above, I found the many pressures and requirements just too annoying and stressful. Looking back on my career it is a miracle that I lasted that long in the clinic! Added to that, the increasing rules and regulations from both Medicare and private insurances were making me grumpy, easily irritated and frustrated. And as I got older the exhausting pace that I had to keep up to maintain my income at somewhat of a predictable level began to wear me down. Medical overhead costs increased at a pace much faster than medical revenues and to keep an even income stream it was necessary to press harder in my work schedule. I suffered from what is now known as "burnout" which is a syndrome effecting physicians that is all too common in our present medical environment affecting as many as 50% or more of physicians at some time or other in their careers. Burnout is characterized by 3 major symptoms: physical, mental and emotional exhaustion; cynicism manifested by a tendency to lose the ability to empathize and connect with your patients, colleagues and loved ones and a tendency to depersonalize your relationships; and doubt that what you are doing really makes any difference at all! Burnout is the main reason why surveys of physicians aged 50 or more show a very high percentage stating that they are actively looking for or at least hoping for something to do other than practice medicine. I started to look around for something else I could do to earn a living, but found that I wasn't really qualified to do anything that would produce an income for me and my family! I was too young and too financially committed to be able to retire. At that personally very dark time I was rescued by an opportunity to be a hospitalist at a small hospital that was only a few miles from my home. So, I said goodbye to my long-term clinic patients and became a hospitalist. As it turned out the change saved my professional life!

The life of a hospitalist is significantly less stressful than that of a clinic based primary care internist. That is why only about 20% of internal medicine doctors are seeking employment in a clinic situation and is why internal medicine primary care doctors are the most highly sought after and recruited specialists presently. It is also a reason why salaries for these physicians are rising even to the point that their earnings from salary may outpace the income they can produce and their salaries are supplemented by the employer physician group. At any rate, I took a position as a hospitalist at a 40-bed long term acute care (LTAC) hospital. Our hospital got all of its patients as referrals from other acute care hospitals. These patients were sick enough to require a prolonged hospital stay—generally 2-4 weeks—and that was financially a drain on the acute care hospital under the DRG payment system. LTACs have a different payment regimen that allows them to take these longer-term patients and still have a positive income profile. I had no exposure to patients needing admission from the ER or from their homes. I was the only full-time hospitalist at the LTAC and was supported by several specialist physicians who consulted there. I also employed a nurse practitioner (NP). My day consisted of daily rounds on the current patients adjusting their treatment regimens and responding to changes in their medical status, admitting new patients to the hospital—usually 2 or 3 a day but at busy times as many as 7 or 8, and some administrative duties. The last several years I was appointed as medical director and had administrative duties as well for which I received a stipend. I was always on call, but since I knew all of the patients and was for the most part able to provide them comprehensive care during the day I only got called when they had a medical status change afterhours. I rarely got more than a few calls, and only had to return to the hospital at night a few times a month. My overhead consisted of the salary I paid to the NP, and some business office charges to code, process and collect my billing. I was an independent contractor and not an employee of the hospital. The burnout issues that I had dealt with in my clinic practice in large part went away and my average work week was 35-40 hours instead of 60! Also, my income increased significantly primarily due to reduced overhead expenses. I happily worked there until I decided to retire. Towards the end there were increasing frustrations again almost exclusively due to changing Medicare rules and regulations that made the administrators more stressed and some of that stress overflowed to me.

Most hospitalists are internal medicine specialists. They are particularly well trained to take care of hospital patients. Today's internal medicine trained doctors are usually ending up about 40% going on to some subspecialty (especially cardiology, or gastroenterology—the high income guys!), 40% to hospitalist practice, and only 20% to outpatient clinic practice. The life of a hospitalist is a pretty good life. They usually work 3-4 twelve hour shifts at the hospital per week, have no "off shift" hospital obligations, and make on average about $200,000 per year. They have no overhead and all they need to do is show up to work with their stethoscope. Some take on administrative assignments, but when they are not at the hospital they have no work issues and are not on call. Some moonlight for extra income, and some just enjoy their time off. They tend to be a bit of a transient group moving from hospital to hospital as they get the urge for new scenery. They are employed by the hospital they work at usually although some are independent hospitalist groups that contract with hospitals. For hospitalists this is the "golden age" of medicine as compared to the office based doctor who sees their golden age very dimly in the rearview mirror! But hospitalist too have their frustrations. Many are now feeling underappreciated and undervalued for the contribution they make to the patient's care in the hospital. This is especially true in the hospitalists interaction with the specialists in the "glamor" fields of cardiology, surgery, and orthopedics from whom the hospitalists feel they get no respect and are treated like "interns". Also, in these days of tightening Medicare rules and regulations with an eye towards decreasing hospital costs, it is upon the shoulders of the hospitalists that the most administrative pressures for controlling costs settle. The "golden age" for hospitalists may end up being relatively short as these hospital cost containment pressures and rules become more mature. Being hospital employees, the hospitalists are subject to increasingly tight management by the hospital administration.

Family and Friends

There is an old adage in medicine: "A physician who treats himself has a fool for a patient!" This kind of flies in the face of the Biblical reference: "Physician, heal thyself" (Luke 4:24). But, the fact of the matter is that doctors make lousy patients and especially so when they are also trying to be their own doctor. They should be in the best position to recognize and identify serious symptoms and be able to make a diagnosis of potentially serious situations very early in the clinical course. But physicians seem to be blind to their own symptoms, and often ignore symptoms thus becoming seriously ill and getting treatment late in the course of the disease. They are also prone to overreact and treat themselves for diseases they do not have. It is a slippery slope for a doctor to have himself as a patient and unfortunately too frequently doctors get in trouble with treatments and medications that they prescribe for themselves. There are many examples of very competent physicians mistreating themselves so badly that they could sue themselves for malpractice! But, that is not what this chapter is about.

Physicians are also not very wise when they treat their family and friends. But it is almost unavoidable. After all, your family are so proud to have a doctor who is related to them that they want you to be the one who diagnoses and treats all their problems. They may go to see other doctors, but will always want to ask you: "My doctor said I had multiple sclerosis, what do you think?" Or they may say: "My doctor gave me a prescription for a statin to take to lower my cholesterol, should I take it?" Or, they may say: "I read about this new treatment for my cancer, do you think I should take it?" You, the physician will get cornered at family reunions, or get phone calls from fairly distant relatives all of whom want to get your opinion about their symptoms, or their disease, or something that their physician diagnosed or some treatment that was prescribed. It doesn't seem to matter to your family that the clinical question they are asking you is outside of the scope of your specialty. It is not in their mind set to realize that their treating physician has access to their actual lab tests, X-ray results, etc. and all you have is their question! They seem to think that all physicians know everything about every disease. It seems inconceivable to them that you—their son, brother, uncle, cousin, etc.—is not up to date on every medical question and treatment, and so, they ask. They don't realize that when they tell you about their "disease" there is left out much pertinent clinical information that they may not know, or do not disclose to you. And, you may not be expert in the treatment of their problem. What do you say to their question? That is why it would be better if every doctor practiced hundreds of miles away from family and friends! My parents, even though I arranged to have them see a very good internist-partner of mine would, without fail, call me after their appointments and ask me what I thought about what their doctor had told them to do. They even often asked me to refill their prescriptions for them. What was I supposed to do—tell them no? So, although my partner was their doctor of record, I was really their physician. This put me in a compromised position. It would have been better if I had just told them: "Go ask your doctor that question!" But I often found myself in a physician-treating-patient position with them.

The situation was not just confined to close family. Uncles, cousins, aunts and more distant relatives would sometimes call me to ask my opinion about their medical condition. Worse than that, I would often get questions about one of their friends who I didn't even know. In those situations, the medical information that was available to me was filtered by their own lack of information and tainted by their own ignorance of the medical problem. First-hand hard medical data was never available to me. Usually, in those situations I just advised them to get back to their treating doctor with their questions. Sometimes I was able to provide them with references to medical specialists that I trusted that might be able to solve their medical dilemma. In my particular situation, I became the treating physician for three of my four grandparents (my other grandfather died before I became a physician, or I would have been his doctor also.) I really didn't want to be their doctor, but every time they had a new problem, or with every new test recommended or treatment ordered they wanted to speak to me first before deciding to proceed. It just became easier for me to be their doctor. Each of my three grandparents eventually became old, feeble and required more and more care. Each of them ended up in a skilled nursing facility ("nursing home") and rather than turn their care over to the "house doctor" who I didn't even know, I remained their physician. Each of them eventually expired under my care and my signature is on their death certificates. In several cases there were hard clinical decisions that needed to be made, including to treat or not to treat, and I bore the responsibility for all of that. Now, I was used to taking responsibility for patient's care, and to attend them through their terminal illnesses and death, but it was much more uncomfortable to be in that position for someone I loved, and under the scrutiny of my close and extended family. It caused me to have much serious reflection trying to be sure that I was not letting my personal and familial feelings jade my medical clinical decision making. In the end, I was grateful to be able to have the skills and experience to help, but I would have preferred to have just been a loving grandson instead.

I was involved in all the details of my parent's medical care. I lived in the same town as them. Both of them ended up in the hospital that I attended at several times with life-threatening illnesses, and I was the first on-scene doctor when those emergency events happened. Of course, I took the lead in helping to stabilize their medical conditions, and I guess it would be right to say that I saved their lives several times. The same held true for my wife's parents. My mother, bless her heart, never seemed to be able to understand that I didn't know all the medical details about every patient who was in the hospital. She would often ask me: "Kirk, my friend LuJean is in the hospital, what is wrong with her and what are you doing to treat it?" To which I just had to answer: "Mom, I'm not taking care of her and I don't even know her and I have no idea about the questions you are asking me about her!" It was hard to try to explain to her that it would not be proper for me to "look in their chart" while I was at the hospital so I could answer her questions about her friend. But that answer never satisfied my mother—I guess I should be proud to think that she felt I was such a good doctor that I should be taking care of every patient in the hospital. Such is the life of a doctor whose family are so proud of him that they cannot imagine anyone would not want to be his patient.

Friends and neighbors present an especially knotty problem. It was not unusual for me to have friends and neighbors just drop in at my home to ask me a medical question about themselves or "someone" that they knew. I could usually deflect those questions pretty well by telling them that I just didn't have enough information about the particulars to be able to answer their question. Sometimes I could give them some education about a particular medical problem or medication or treatment, but I would be able to leave it at that. Sometimes they wanted a "second opinion" and I had to point out to them that they were not providing me with enough medical data to be able to do that properly. The bigger problem was when they were wanting me to treat them. They would often begin the conversation with: "Kirk, I didn't want to bother you at the office but I have a problem I wanted to ask you about!" When I was especially grouchy I would tell them: "Make an appointment to come see me at the office—that is where I go to be bothered by people's medical problems", but I always felt that way in my mind! Most of the time I was able to avoid the booby-trap of treating them out of my house with inadequate examination and medical testing and no medical record being generated. It was not about getting paid for my services, but was about the medical liability that I took on if I informally treated my neighbor or friend and made a serious error due to inadequate information. In my neighborhood, I had an herbalist and a person who was a proponent of "essential oils". Not infrequently my neighbor was there with the question about their symptoms and the statement: "Mike told me to do take this herb, and Jen told me use this essential oil, what do you think?" I always answered that question with: "Go see a doctor!"

My wife and I were married through my medical training and my medical practice. We often talked about medical things and I think that she assumed that she had a store of medical information from our conversations. She is a loving and caring person and sincerely wants to help others. It was not uncommon that I would be home and hear my wife in conversation on the phone, and notice that the conversation was clearly medical in nature with my wife providing advice and recommendations! It even happened that occasionally I would be the one who answered the phone and the person on the other end of the line would be surprised that I was on the line, then after a pause ask to talk to my wife. Subsequently I would overhear that the conversation was about medical things! Our friends or neighbors were using my wife as a surrogate doctor! I often told her that she was "practicing medicine without a license", but she just couldn't seem to help herself. Such abuse of friendship and neighborliness is, I am sure, the common lot of all physicians. Some physicians just bruskly refuse to be involved in these conversations. Other's like me end up being put in very uncomfortable situations. I was often asked by my church group to do "physicals" for the Boy Scouts in our local troop for summer camp as well as for the young women for their church sponsored activities. How do you say no to that? But, I advised all the parents that my "home" version of a physical consisted only of a medical history, a blood pressure and listening to their hearts…. if they wanted a better physical than that they needed to go see their personal family doctor. I even got dragged in to doing physicals for the adult leader, against my better judgement. But, having opened the door and agreeing to do Scout physicals led to many of the neighbors to ask if I would do the high school sports physicals for their children. That made me even more uncomfortable, given the liability that could be incurred if a serious medical problem was missed by my cursory examination. After many years I just stopped agreeing to these requests and I think my neighbors were not satisfied with the reason I gave for stopping.

    Of course, I treated my children for their simple infections, lacerations, strains and sprains and injuries. No need to go to their pediatrician and spend money on a medical visit when I was perfectly capable of providing their care. But, I did not want my children to become medical neurotics always wanting some medicine or treatment for their colds or other minor, self-limited problems. Maybe I went too far in that directions. When they hurt themselves I would give them very little sympathy telling them that "It will feel better when it stops hurting!" Or, I would often tell them that they didn't need to worry about this cut or sprain since "It is a long way from your heart!" We refused to put bandages on "sunshine sores", and told them, "no, you don't need to go see the doctor for that simple problem." I often brought them to my office all together to have them get their flu shots in the fall. If you ask them they will all say that they hated that. I had some basic medical equipment at home and sewed up their simple lacerations on the kitchen table. I drained my oldest son's cauliflower ear that he got from wrestling in high school without his head gear on. I even sewed up one of their cousins when he got a laceration while at our house at a family gathering with all of my children and their cousins watching on in horrible fascination! I gave my number two son his allergy shots for hay fever at home, rather than have my wife take him to the allergist twice a week for several years. At the occasion of the first allergy shot, he said to me "Dad, have you ever done this before?" Actually, no, I had never given allergy shots before but was sure that I was capable of doing it, so I told him "yes, son, lots of times." I even sewed up a few of the neighbor children whose parents brought them over to "see if they needed stitches". Such is your life if you are a physician-husband-father-relative-neighbor.

Playing Well With Others

The story is told of two doctors, one a surgeon and one an internist, who went duck hunting together. Some birds were seen in the distance and Bang! the surgeon fired quickly saying: "A duck, at least I thought it was a duck, for sure it was a duck, that's what I am going to report---it was a duck!" The internist saw the same flock of birds but as it was going by he held his fire saying: "those look like ducks, are they mallards or are they mergansers, but then again, loons like kind of like that, I don't think they are geese, I need to consider this a minute to be sure I don't shoot a bird that is not in season!" as the flock flies out of sight. This story is an illustration of the differences in mental mind set and approach to patients that you will see as you get to know doctors of different specialties. Surgeons are often heard to say: "a chance to cut is a chance to cure" or "nothing cannot be fixed with the proper application of a Bard Parker scalpel blade!" Internists on the other hand are all about differential diagnosis, tests to confirm the diagnosis and careful and methodical treatment of the patient. They want to be sure they are exact in their diagnosis and prudent in their treatment of the patient. You will find if you get to know a number of doctors in different specialties that there are some typical personalities that seem to gravitate in the various specialty fields of medicine. Of course, there are exceptions and sometimes you will find a surgeon with and internist's careful methodical approach to patient care, or an internist who seems to fire of a diagnosis almost instantly. I am not sure whether the personality type before medical school drives some physicians to some specialties (probably does to some extent) or whether the training and experience practicing one of the specialties molds the personality of the physician (there is likely an element of this.) But you have a bunch of medical practitioners all with their own personalities and approaches to patient care often sharing in the treatment of individual patients. In the ideal world these various physicians would "play well together" but that is not so often the case.

The buzz phrase in medical care today is "collaborative care". By that is meant that a variety of health care providers—physicians of different specialties, NPs and PAs, nurses, physical therapists, pharmacists, etc.—should work together cooperatively to treat the patient. In studies that have looked at this type of collaboration there is evidence that the patient does in fact benefit from this approach. The problem is that those studies have looked at treatment teams that are assembled for the pre-stated purpose of doing collaborative care. In the real world of medical practice that is rarely the situation. In the real world the physicians and health care professionals that treat the patient are not consciously a team and each comes to the patient with their own set of skills and knowledge making treatment recommendations or providing treatment with their own specialty focus in mind. Patients often go from specialist to specialist for consultation and the various specialists "do their thing" without much consideration for the "thing" that the other doctors are doing to or for the total patient. Even when the patient is in the hospital and the specialists come to them, each doctor focuses on the "thing" that is their part of the patient without much thought at all to the other parts. What happens then is fragmented care, not collaborative care. This leads often to repeated tests, redundant or excessive medications with possible unanticipated medication interactions, and a patient who is confused about just what exactly is wrong with them. And the cost of medical care is multiplied by this multitude of physician care providers. It is a rare thing indeed in my experience when all of the doctors literally or figuratively "sit down together" and discuss the patient as a whole to decide what a unified treatment plan should be. The closest I ever came to this was my days as a hospitalist at the LTAC where we sat together weekly as a treatment team to coordinate the care of each patient. In that setting I was usually the only physician or maybe we would have a consultant doctor as well on the patient's case.

In day to day medical care situations that involve one patient and multiple treating physicians it is usually the case that there is confusion about "who is in charge here?" Each physician is often quite insistent about their treatment recommendations based upon the "piece" of the patient that fits into their specialty area and conflicts can arise between doctors when other treating physicans change the treatment plan, medication, orders for testing, etc. The poor patient is often left with a long list of medications, an expensive set of diagnostic tests ordered, and all the time thinking that the doctors are surely talking to each other about their individual medical care when in fact that is not happening. Surely this problem accounts for a significant portion of the expense of medical care and at times it leads to patient harm.

I have always felt like I wanted to keep the number of other doctors who were treating my patients to a minimum. The old culinary adage that "too many cooks spoil the pot" is true in medical care as well. Ideally, the patient has a physician who takes the view that they are responsible for the total patient and makes sure that all of the care given by other doctors is appropriate, timely and not conflicting. Unfortunately, the best physician for that job is a good family physician or internist. The reason that is unfortunate is because the family physician or internist is often viewed by other medical specialists as a lower-class citizen of the medical social strata. It is pretty stressful for an internist to confront a surgeon, or a cardiologist, or a gastroenterologist, or other specialty physician and question the care given or the recommendations made by that specialist. Not only is it stressful, but it is often unsuccessful as these specialists consider themselves the authority figure in the conversation. And, once a specialist makes a recommendation and stands by it the generalist doctor is put in a potential liability position if those recommendations are not followed even if they feel the best interests of the patient are not served. Doctors are intelligent, opinionated, hard-working and busy and they often do not play well together. I wish it was otherwise!

A big problem that derives from this involves the payment for medical care. Private insurances often try to reduce the expense of medical care by assigning a generalist physician as the "primary care physician" (PCP). This physician is supposed to coordinate the care of the patient especially in view of other specialty physicians who may see the patient. Often the PCP is a "gate-keeper" and is supposed to be consulted by the patient to authorize a visit to a specialist before the patient can go see them. HMO insurance plans actually put the PCP at financial risk if they overspend the insurance budget by sending patients to specialists too often, or if the tests and procedures provided by specialists exceeds a budgeted amount of money. Medicare has embraced a concept called "medical home" which is essentially the same concept applied to Medicare patients. But in the real world most specialists are not very likely to take direction from a generalist physician or ask the generalist physician whether or not it would be alright to do a test or procedure. When physicians know each other well and have a long standing working relationship this may work fairly well, but in the more usual situation where the physicians don't have any kind of personal experience with each other it falls quickly apart.

Now adding to the problem of "playing together well" are new Medicare initiatives and rules aimed at reducing the costs of medical care. One is the Accountable Care Organization (ACO). In an ACO a group of physicians associate together and have a number of Medicare patients assigned to them for the purposes of managing expenses. The patients don't know they are assigned to an ACO and the doctors in the ACO may not have a long working relationship with each other. If the ACO can deliver care to these patients at less than the historical cost then they get to share financially in the savings, but if their ACO provides care at greater than the historical cost then they are financially penalized. A recent report of outcomes with ACOs showed several groups did have some savings, but viewed as a whole—all the ACOs together—no Medicare savings was realized. It is really hard for physicans to play together well unless they are tightly managed….and there is the rub. Doctors don't like to be managed, and especially not by non-MDs! Another approach to make physicians "play well together" for the purpose of managing the cost of providing care is the proposed Medicare plan to "bundle" payment on hospitalized patients. This would pay a set amount from Medicare to the hospital for the total care of the patient including physician care and then require the hospital and the physicians to negotiate what proportion of the money is "theirs". They would have to agree how to divide up the monetary pie in the most equitable way considering the relative contribution each party played in taking care of the patient. Now, this plan might work if physicians did "play well together" but when it comes to splitting up the money do not expect to see a reasoned and peaceful interaction. When it comes to getting paid doctors are not very collaboratively minded. I remember a patient that I took care of who had multiple complications after a hip replacement. These complications led to some time in the ICU and a few weeks' total in the hospital. The orthopedic surgeon spent about 2 hours' total replacing the hip and I spent easily 5 times that amount of time managing the complications. When I made a comment to the orthopedist that he likely made 5 times what I did taking care of that patient his not so understanding reply was: "Well, if you wanted to make what an orthopedic surgeon makes you should have gone into orthopedics!" So much for a collaborative mind set.

In the ideal world all medical care would be collaborative. Each doctor or health care practitioner would view the patient from a holistic perspective. Each would consider whether the treatment rendered by them would interfere with the treatment rendered by other members of the treatment team. The doctors would actually talk together about the patient to work out the details of a comprehensive treatment plan that all could support. And there would be one physician assigned to be the one to coordinate and manage the patient's medical care, and the patient would know who that physician was. All patient information would be instantly available to each member of the treatment team. This ideal world does not exist! It doesn't have much chance of becoming the reality in the current dysfunctional medical care system we have in the USA. Whether or not a new collaborative paradigm could live inside the coming medical care system in the USA is questionable. Unless it is seen as the primary goal of the new system it is unlikely to see any life in the future. If it is not planned for, it will not happen.

The Digital Age

    Time was in the past that a doctor made notes about his patients for the purpose of reminding the doctor of the patient's medical problems, treatments that had been prescribed, and how the patient responded to the treatments. Every doctor developed their own system of notations that made sense to them in fulfilling these needs. These were not the patient's medical records, but were the physician's notes regarding their patients. Insurance companies never saw these notes, government agencies never saw these notes, even other doctors didn't see these notes. The notes were all hand written and contained a lot of abbreviations and Latin and Greek symbols that had medical or notational meaning. Doctor's written prescriptions were particularly hard to decipher and contained notations that were intelligible to the doctor and the pharmacist but to very few others. Doctor's handwriting has been a source of jokes for years and rightly so. I have often joked with people about this when I have told them that the first part of any student's application to medical school is a brief essay and if the admission committee can read it then that application is put in the "not for admission" pile! Not so in reality but doctors are notoriously poor at penmanship. Early in my practice I was associated with several physicians that were 20 plus years my senior and their patient notes in the patient chart were unintelligible. On more than one occasion I had seen one of my partner's patients while he was away and I was on call and after looking at the chart from every point on the compass just had to resort to asking the patient what problems they were being treated for and with what medications. Even a day or two later if I had occasion to ask that particular physician to interpret what he had written in his notes he was unable to do so with precision! Thus was the state of the patient's medical records even up in to the 1980s and beyond.

    When I was in medical school we students were taught some systems of medical record keeping in an attempt to standardize notations in a way that would be uniform across the profession. Outlines for recording the elements of the patient history and physical exam were pressed upon us. This was a good thing since it helped to have necessary patient medical information always noted in a fairly standardized way so that any doctor might be able to make sense out of what was there. In the 1970s Dr. Lawrence Weed attempted to bring order and standardization to the problem of medical record keeping. He developed and promoted the "problem oriented medical record" and with it the "SOAP" note pattern of medical notation. SOAP stands for the 4 elements of the problem oriented medical note: "Subjective"—what the patient tells the doctor; "Objective"—what the doctor sees when the patient is examined or with lab or x-rays, etc.; "Assessment"—what the doctor's diagnosis is; and "Plan"—what the prescribed course of action is that the doctor is going to recommend. This system was taught to me in medical school, but some of my senior partners in my private practice never adopted the system. Their notes were just one continuous paragraph of unreadable notation that somehow expressed the essence of the patient-physician interaction. The SOAP note was not just a notation system but it served as a framework for medical assessment and planning and guided the physician's thinking and assessment process. For the first 20 plus years of my medical practice all of my patient notes where hand written in the Weed format and it served me well enough and my other partners could make sense of my medical decision making if they had occasion to see one of my patients in my absence.

Things started to change when insurance companies and government started to feel that since they were paying the bills they wanted to be able to review what was done by the doctor. Medical records were requested and reviewed and often payments were withheld or modified based on the 3rd party's interpretation. With the advent of "managed care" insurance plans the medical records were often reviewed to determine whether the insurance company would "preauthorize" some test or procedure. Increasing detail was required in the medical notes to provide documentation of the patient's need. After a while, the medical record was also scrutinized to determine what level of care was provided to see if it justified the physicians bill—the ICD and CPT codes had increasingly detailed criterion for each diagnosis and procedure code that had to be included in the physician's notes to justify payment of the physician's fee. Physicians soon learned what information was necessary to be in a medical note to justify the level of billing that they submitted to the insurance company. Doctors aren't stupid so when faced with the need for certain information in their note, even if felt to be non-pertinent to the patient's care, physicians learned how to "polish" up their notes to meet the expectation and produce the payment desired. A whole new regulatory industry was formed to review medical records for regulatory and payment purposes. Physician overhead costs increased because most doctors moved from hand written notes to dictated notes that required transcription. A physician's time was increasingly spent producing the medical record—time that either took away from direct patient care time, or added significant physician time in addition to the time they spent doing direct patient care. Some physicians hired "scribes" to free them from medical record keeping—the scribe attended the physician/patient visit and made all the notations. Of course, only the high earning physicians can afford this luxury. Some physicians became especially adept at "polishing" the medical record including all the elements the regulators wanted to see even if it made no difference in how the patient was taken care of. It seemed that the regulators were more interested in what was in the medical record than how the patient really was doing with their treatment. "Quality of care" assessments were made by the 3rd parties based upon elements that were included in the medical record. Doctors started to "doctor" the medical records as much or more than they "doctored" the patient.

   Then came the digital age. Like almost everything else in our modern lives this transformed medical practice. CT scans, MRI's, digital color flow ultrasound, PET scans and a host of medical technologies became available with digital technology. So it was with the medical record as well. Many businesses sprang up providing digital software for medical record keeping. Each company used their own formatted software and from my perspective produced digital "templates" designed by software engineers who knew nothing about how doctors think, notate or document their services. Some digital programs were pretty good but demanded quite a lot of time by the physician to learn how to use them. But now there is still problems with "interoperability"—each proprietary program is unique and they don't interconnect so that digital notes in one program just turn out to be nonsense when transmitted to some other program. Medical records cannot be transmitted electronically between different software platforms. The promise of "paperless" medical record keeping has not been realized. In my work as a hospitalist I had occasion to review medical records from many hospitals each using different digital software programs and found a frustratingly wide array of formats that took time to navigate to find the desired information. And these digital software programs are expensive with costs for a one-man physician office approaching $50,000 for software and hardware! Larger medical groups get some economies of scale but even then, large healthcare providers like hospital systems and large physician clinics can easily spend tens of millions for an Electronic Medical Record (EMR) system. The digitization of the medical record has just added another significant amount to the physician's financial overhead expense. And most physicians surveyed report that up to 40% of their work time is taken up with just producing the medical record! This reduces the time available to spend with direct patient interaction and care.

Now enter Medicare into the system. First Medicare established rules for electronic submission of physician bills for payment. Target dates for implementation were set and penalties were applied for non-compliance. All physician offices and hospitals had to comply or not be paid! Second, Medicare established rules and dates for accomplishment requiring electronic medical record (EMR) usage by all physicians and hospitals. Again, target dates for implementation and penalties were applied for non-compliance with a reduction of 1% from Medicare payments for those physicians who missed the deadlines. "Meaningful Use" rules were put in place in a 3-stage process that pushed physicians towards total use of EMR. The stated purpose for this was to allow for standardized documentation of medical care so as to allow Medicare to be able to review the record and measure Medicare defined "quality metrics" that will eventually result in payment penalties for physician non-compliance. "Quality of care" was defined by the inclusion of certain elements in the medical note, and not by how the patient was actually doing clinically! (You have heard about the surgeon who told the family that the surgery went well, but the patient died! Well, the EMR can show that the care met "quality" standards but the patient didn't do so well. Most doctors feel that the emphasis on the comprehensive EMR is actually taking away from the quality of physician delivered health care.) The eventual use of the EMR by Medicare will be used to determine whether or not to reimburse the physician their full (Medicare approved) fee for patient care or to withhold a percentage of the fee due to failure of meeting quality metric standards. The medical profession is in an uproar about these requirements. Phase 3 implementation rules and dates have been pushed back due to complaints. As I have stated before: if Medicare had set out with the overtly stated purpose to make as many doctors refuse to take care of Medicare patients as possible they could not have done a better job! Eventually this will all get worked out but this is just another factor that adds to the very long list of physician's complaints about the red tape and expense that is involved in taking care of their patients in the current regulatory milieu. Patients don't seem to like it either. They are not aware of all the stresses and expenses the EMR is causing their doctors. What they are aware of serves as one of their most common complaints about their interaction with their doctors: "My doctor spends more time looking at the computer than he does listening to me!" The EMR is depersonalizing the patient-physician relationship even while it is attempting to improve the "quality" of medical care by demanding digitally measured patient care outcomes documentation. Oh, the age we live in! And on top of this, doctors universally report that using an EMR adds 1.5 or more hours to their work day. Surely the time is near at hand when the entire patient's personal medical record will be able to be reduced to a small memory device like a "thumb drive" (or maybe even an implantable "chip") and become completely portable, universally accessible and able to be downloaded by any health provider or hospital. This will be valuable, but for now the EMR is just a source of frustration for physicians and a major contributor to physician burn out.

And while on the topic of the digital age I must be sure to make a comment about how the internet has effected the practice of medicine. The internet is a blessing and a curse! That is true for most aspects of it and is surely true for the medical aspects. Patients can now look up their symptoms and make their own diagnosis on the internet. Most of this time they are in error because the average person is unable to sort the true from the erroneous on the internet. Many people seem to believe that "someone" is in control of the internet and if you read something there it has been vetted to assure that it is true! But there is truth on the internet and especially the younger generations of patients now regularly come to the doctor's appointment already sure of what they "have" and what they "need" and they become immediately suspicious of the doctor if the physician does not agree with the preconceived diagnosis of their symptoms. And worse possibly than that, as soon as the patient leaves the doctor's visit they look up what the doctor prescribed to see if they will believe the advice and counsel they have been given. Although the internet has the opportunity to strengthen the compliance of the patient with the physician's prescription, it often serves to weaken it instead. Patients read about "side effects" of medications and then refuse to take them because the side effects seem worse than the disease that was diagnosed. Internet patient portals are now available from hospitals and larger medical clinics that allow the patient to access their own medical records including labs, x-rays and pathology reports at any time providing the patient the data to make their own interpretations and diagnosis. No longer will the doctor be able just to say "all your tests are normal" without the patient also being able to actually see the test results on line. Conversely the physician will be at risk of having their diagnosis "second guessed" by the patient who reviews their own medical data. And now add another new wrinkle in the practice of medicine— "telemedicine". Medical clinics and other medical vendor organizations are offering virtual doctor's appointments over a secured internet connection. These interactions are now being recognized by insurance providers and being paid for by them. This is in its infancy but expect to see this kind of service blossom in the next decade as it has the promise of offering physician services at all times of day and night and without the need of appointment, travel, waiting time, etc. Also, it solves the digital dilemma for the doctor—they can look at the computer screen and the patient thinks that they are looking at them! Now instead of a negative, the digitalization of the medical encounter becomes a positive. Expect to see software "apps" become available that will allow the patient to input vital signs information like temperature, heart rate, respiratory rate, and blood pressure during the virtual encounter, and even at some time even higher tech digital probes that will allow for other data to be gathered by the physician during this virtual doctor's visit. Is the time really coming that a physician can use a Star Trek like "Tricorder" applied remotely over an internet application to make a diagnosis and provide treatment to the patient? Don't doubt it for a moment!

     Finally, on the topic of the digitalization of medicine I have to comment upon the privacy aspects of the medical record. The Health Information Portability and Accountability Act (HIPAA) of 1996 established laws that protect the privacy of the medical records of individuals. This act sets very strict rules governing the privacy of medical records. It specifies under what circumstances and to whom medical information about a particular patient can be shared. It provides fines and criminal penalties for violations of its regulations. As our medical encounters become more digital, virtual and electronic there will need to be new security features developed to keep them private. There have been many publicized personal data breeches with credit cards and social security numbers and the like already. The criminals always seem to be ahead of the game on this. The more we have our personal medical data digitally rendered the more the possibility will be for it to be "hacked". Not only will breeches of privacy be possible for those with criminal intent, but also by those who have other motivations including departments of government and corporations who seek information to promote their business or to screen potential clients or employees. And, like with Facebook and other internet based programs, medical information could be used by marketers to target specific medical populations to which they can advertise and promote their products and services. Great caution will need to be exercised as this venture proceeds to mature. Additionally, there is now a real unanswered question of who the medical record belongs to—does it belong to the physician, the patient or the insurance company that is paying for the care? What do you think?

Malpractice

The practice of medicine is risky business…both for the doctor as well as for the patient. There are many illnesses that are fatal if not treated, or that lead to significant disability. Medical and surgical treatments have been developed to treat these serious maladies but the treatments themselves are associated with the risk of untoward consequences. Despite many "miraculous" cures that have been developed everyone eventually succumbs to the one condition that is not curable: mortality. The art and practice of medicine is not yet perfect, and it is administered by the hands of imperfect and often severely stressed human physicians. No treatment yet devised is 100% effective and 100% safe. An example: a statistical construct that is used to assess a new medical treatment is the "number needed to treat" (NNT) which is a description of how many patients with a particular illness must be treated with a particular treatment in order to have one favorable outcome. That favorable outcome might be one less heart attack than expected in the group that was treated with a statin for hypercholesterolemia. For statin treatment in persons who did not have known heart disease the NNT is 104—you must treat 104 persons without known heart disease with statins to prevent one heart attack that would have occurred. In patients with known heart disease the NNT is 39—you must treat 39 to prevent one heart attack that would otherwise have occurred. That would be pretty good if it weren't for the fact that up to 29% of persons who take statins develop muscle pain or muscle inflammation, a few percentages develop liver inflammation, a small percentage may develop diabetes or memory problems with statins. Even in the face of these facts it is essentially universally recommended by physicians to treat patients with statins to prevent heart attack and stroke. Although we know that we can prevent one heart attack per every 39 people treated, we cannot predict which person of the 39 will be the one spared, nor can we predict which 11 people (29% of 39) will be the ones who develop muscle problems related to the statin. If we were to compute the NNH (number needed to harm—how many patients need to be treated with this particular therapy to result in 1 bad outcome) for statins it would be 3.5 (39 divided by 11). But the side effects of statins are much less serious than a heart attack! This example can be multiplied by the 100s—maybe thousands-- for all of the other medications and surgical treatments that physicians administer to patients daily. When it comes down to it the practice of medicine is to apply treatments that will do the best for the most people while reducing the harm done to the least number of patients. As I said, the practice of medicine can be hazardous to both the patient and the doctor—to the doctor who gets sued for prescribing the right medication or treatment to an appropriate patient but ends up with an untoward effect that cannot be blamed on the doctor's incompetence!

     A recently highly publicized report was made in the British Medical Journal (BMJ 2016:353, May 2016) sensationally claiming that medical errors were the 3rd leading cause of death in the USA accounting for 250,000 deaths per year. Cancer and heart disease are numbers 1 and 2 with about 600,000 deaths per year. But a flaw in the study was the manner in which medical errors were defined: *"Medical error has been defined as an unintended act (either of omission or commission) or one that does not achieve its intended outcome, or the failure of a planned action to be completed as intended (an error of execution), or the use of a wrong plan to achieve an aim (an error of planning), or a deviation from the process of care that may or may not cause harm to the patient."*

It essentially defines as one example of a medical error the unplanned occurrence of a death due to the application of a medical treatment.   Or it also defined as a medical error a death due to the failure to apply a treatment.   So, in this definition a medical error (though not a fatal one) would be the muscle pain that occurred in 11/39 people treated with a statin even though one may have been spared a heart attack. It would also define as a medical error the failure to prescribe a statin to a 95-year-old person with known heart disease even though that elderly person would have better than 30% chance of suffering from side effects of the statin and only a 1/39 chance of avoiding a heart attack because of the medication. In surgical treatments there are well established expected death or significant untoward effects of each type of surgery. If a person has a surgery that was done properly but dies is that really a "medical error" if the surgical mortality rate of that particular procedure of 2% (for example) means that 2 people will die with the surgery for every 100 people operated on? The point of all of this is that the term "malpractice" as it is used in the USA does not imply that the doctor did something wrong but that things didn't turn out as well as the patient and the doctor expected. This is an unreasonable and unattainable standard to ask of medical practitioners. The doctor is a looser in every scenario if the standard is to provide the proper service properly delivered to the proper patient 100% of the time and have 0% complications and a 100% success rate! Even God might not be able to do that well.

You can't turn on the TV during prime time without seeing adds placed by attorneys advertising for patients that were "harmed" by some medication or surgical treatment. The legal culture in the US is such that anything less than a 100% favorable outcome with a 100% absence of untoward effects is the only acceptable end point for patient care. Because of these malpractice allegations are made against physicians with alarming frequency. An estimated 17,000 malpractice suits are filed against physicians in the USA yearly. But 78% of the claims fail to result in payments to the patients and if the case goes to a jury trial the physician is vindicated 85-90% of the time by a jury. 7.4% of all doctors get sued each year with some specialties getting sued at a much higher rate: 19% of neurosurgeons and cardiac surgeons, 15% of general surgeons for example. At that rate the average doctor may get sued 2-3 times or more in their practice lifetime. An average neurosurgeon may get sued 6 or more times. Additionally, hospitals and pharmaceutical companies are frequent targets of malpractice suits. Even when a drug has a known possible side effect, patients may sue in class action suits with the hope of recovering a large cash award. The legal tort system in the USA has been in favor of malpractice legal action and the fact that the attorney's fees usually represent 30% or more of the cash award is highly motivational to personal injury attorneys. Of course, there are times when doctors really have made errors that have resulted in patient harm. Some doctors are careless, or sloppy in their work, some are rude or dismissive of patient's complaints, some are insufficiently educated for the treatment they are providing. Heck, most doctors are all of these things on their worst days! Doctors are human and prone to all of the frailties of the race. But most malpractice suits do not involve real harm and in my experience are more designed to punish the doctor for having prescribed a treatment that did not have the intended favorable outcome even though the treatment was properly prescribed or applied. There seems that there must be a better way to compensate patients who are harmed by the application of modern medical practice to their medical issues than subjecting the treating physician to the process of a malpractice proceeding.

Malpractice allegations usually catch the physician by surprise. Every doctor knows when they have had a difficult case which did not turn out as well as hoped. Most doctors really extend themselves in these cases to try to achieve a positive outcome. They spend time with the patient and family and suffer with them. Only the most sociopathic doctor will not have self-doubt and introspection when these cases happen. But the nature of the US tort system is that there is a 5-year statute of limitations and most patient's or their families take some time to decide to make a malpractice claim, so it is often that the events are 1-2 or more years in the past when the doctor gets the dreaded "intent to sue" notification. Hopefully the medical records available will be sufficient to allow for an accurate portrayal of the actual facts of the case. Plaintiff's attorneys ask detailed questions of what the doctor "remembers" about the case which by the time it gets to deposition time may have been 3-4 years in the past. The wise doctor must not speculate about what they might remember, and must answer "I don't remember" when asked a question that is not documented in the medical record. "I don't remember" is always suspected as an attempt to hide information. How many lay people can remember details of a specific day or two that was 3-4 years ago and was only one of multiple events of a similar nature on that very day? The discovery process and the deposition process in the tort proceeding is such that any inconsistency in the wording of a physician's answer to a question gets more attention by the plaintiff's attorney than any political candidate's stupid comments do on the evening news! So not only is the physician obligated to remember specific details about events far in the past but they must also remember what the exact wording of their answer was to the same question as long as a year or more prior to the deposition when similar questions were answered in the discovery part of the proceeding! The plaintiff's attorney often asks the same question multiple times with minor variation until they are able to leave the physician no option than to give them the answer they want. Speaking from my own experience this is the most unpleasant experience imaginable. The plaintiff's attorney wants to catch the physician in his own words and convict them by their own statements! The question has been asked: is it all right to just have the physician tell the patient or the family that they are "sorry" for how things turned out? You would think that would be best, but the plain fact is that the plaintiff's attorney would use that sympathetic expression of the physician's humanity as the rope to hang them with…why would you be sorry if you did nothing wrong? A doctor who gets sued is almost always not a "bad" doctor, but they are a doctor who took on a difficult case (or even just an average case like hyperlipidemia) that did not turn out as well as everyone hoped it would. But given my discussion above it should be clear to you that every doctor has many cases that do not turn out as well as hoped and it is not due to incompetence on the part of the physician. And patient noncompliance with treatment regimens or preexisting self-imposed health risks (like smoking that leads to heart disease) increase the likelihood of untoward outcomes but is never taken into consideration when a tort proceeding is trying to "blame" the doctor for a less than wonderful medical result.

    The lay person most often hears of malpractice verdicts against doctors when the case is sensational or when the case results in multi-million-dollar pay outs. But most malpractice cases are settled out of court, or are dropped because the plaintiff's attorney decides that the amount of the settlement (their 30% cut) will not cover their costs of prosecuting the case. Some are dropped because on further inspection there was no cause for accusation in the first place. The average malpractice verdict or settlement is $250,000 to $300,000 and that doesn't end up being big news for the public. Personal injury tort practice is such in the USA that the patient doesn't owe the plaintiff's attorney any money if the case does not end in a cash settlement or jury imposed cash verdict. So patients and their families who are suit-minded have nothing to lose in giving it a try if they can find an attorney to take the case. The attorney on the other hand has to lay out significant cash to prosecute the case and if they judge it will not pay them back with profit in the end then they will not take the case. You would think that would result in the plaintiff's attorney taking more care to get educated about the medical facts pertinent to the case, but in the cases I have been personally involved in that has not been the rule. It is my opinion that most plaintiff's attorneys hope that the amount of legal harassment they apply to the doctor in the early course of the proceedings will lead the doctor to instruct their liability insurer to make a cash offer to settle the case just to make it go away. Sometimes too the malpractice insurance company makes a judgement that the costs of defending the case all the way through a trial exceed what the plaintiff might accept in an offer of a cash settlement. So, when a case is settled "out of court" there is no admission or implication of guilt or fault on the part of the physician. Bullying pays in the tort system! It is legalized theft on the plaintiff's part. As I noted above, when the physician stands up to the accusations and takes the charges completely through the trial system the overwhelming majority of cases are decided in the doctor's favor.

    I have been personally sued for malpractice several times. One time ended in a cash settlement because the two other physicians named with me decided to make a cash settlement leaving me as the sole physician on the hot seat if we went to court. My malpractice insurer and attorney recommended the cash settlement rather than subject ourselves to the trial as the sole defendant. I still feel like I was robbed and raped! It was a difficult case involving a young man who developed herpes encephalitis which diagnosis was missed at the first hospital (the other 2 doctors involved) and was diagnosed and started on appropriate treatment by me within 24 hours of admission to the hospital that I was the "on call" doctor for and thus accepted the patient in transfer from the first hospital. This patient went on to develop life threating complications which I was closely monitored him for and for which immediate treatment was applied when they occurred that saved his life. However, he was left with some residual neurological problems when he recovered. Herpes encephalitis has a high death rate and essentially all survivors have some persistent neurological issues so the outcome was as good as it could have been. But the legalized theft allowed by the tort system paid him for his trouble. The other case was clearly not meritorious. An unfortunate elderly female in poor general health had a knee replacement with multiple complications. I became her physician when she was transferred to the LTAC at which I was the attending hospitalist. She subsequently developed pneumonia, acute respiratory failure and died. I was accused of improper treatment and delay in diagnosis. I refused to allow the insurance company to make a cash settlement and went through the indignity of a court trial. The week of the court proceedings was hellish and I lost 10 pounds and slept little. I was on the witness stand for more than half of the entire court time being grilled by the plaintiff's attorney who I came to despise. In the end the jury came to a "not guilty" verdict in less than 30 minutes' deliberation. A week later a family representative met me in the hallway of the LTAC and apologized for putting me through the whole thing stating that they really didn't want to sue me but the attorney they consulted thought that they could win some big money with the case!

You might ask how does it affect a physician to be sued for malpractice? I can only speak for myself but I am sure my feelings are shared by most doctors. The first feeling is unpleasant surprise! You always know that such a thing is a possibility—it is part of the modern practice of medicine. But like most of us you never really thought it would happen to you. You're a good doctor who cares for your patients and tries to do the very best for them. The next feeling is severe anger and rage—how dare they sue me for doing the best that I could to treat their difficult medical condition! I did nothing wrong! That feeling of rage quickly dissolves into severe anxiety caused by self-doubt and second guessing that rapidly progresses to depression. You lose your appetite. You don't sleep well and you play the scenario over and over in your head. You are always just a little bit distracted. You wonder if you really did goof up. All the while you must continue to take care of your patients even when you are suffering from the most acute self-doubt. It clearly changes how you view each patient who comes under your care—are they going to sue you if things don't turn out as they expect? You become hyper-vigilant and suspicious of the motives of your patients. You do things to try to make sure that you "don't miss anything"—yes you may order extra tests or consultations that are not really needed and that you would not have done before. You check and double check that your insurance will cover the cost of any settlement so that you don't lose your house or have to declare bankruptcy. Are you going to end up on the news? Is your reputation going to be ruined? Now this would be bad enough if it went on for weeks or maybe months, but the average malpractice case takes about 2.5 years on average from the initial filing until resolution. During that time, you are subjected to seemingly endless legal questions from your attorney and subjected to hearings and depositions of a very unfriendly nature involving the plaintiff's attorney. Contrary to what the attorneys may say, it is personal—extremely personal! It is a referendum on your competence as a physician and as a human being. You just get some control over the roller coaster of your emotions and self-doubt when they resurface again with each additional new installment of the proceedings. And if you end up going to trial expect to have the worst days of your entire life! I often wondered to myself: why would any sane individual go into a profession where they would be subjected to this kind of personal stress piled on top of the stress already intrinsic to their occupation? Why indeed! In what universe does the practice of medicine pay well enough to compensate for this? What other honorable occupation subjects its practitioners to such abuse as a part of their routine activities? Even when the conclusion to the issue ends in your favor you feel violated. You feel like you would like to sue the plaintiffs and their attorney but that is not allowed in the current Tort system. Even if you get an apology like I did after the trial I went through it is hollow and meaningless. You are less of a person because of what happened. The joy you got out of practicing medicine seems counterfeit. You would quit being a doctor if you had the option, but most of the time you are not rich enough to do that and you are not qualified for any other line of work, so you forge on ahead and try to forget the pain and learn whatever lesson was there for you in the experience. You try to regain a feeling of trust and compassion towards your patients. Like most bad experiences in life, the cure comes with the passage of time...but then again with the average doctor having an 8% chance of being sued each year just as the pain is fading away in your rear view mirror, here it comes again! I ask you, do you as the American public want to have your doctor be affected in all of those ways as they take care of your health issues?

On my good days I remember that I saw an average of 25 patients daily, about 120 per week for 48 weeks a year for a total of 35 years. That represents a total of over 200,000 patient care encounters in my practice career! On balance, and despite the strain that the malpractice experiences caused, I feel that I did a lot of good for these patients. I continually run into former patients of mine who always say "we miss you" and often say "our new doctor just isn't a good to us as you were"! There is satisfaction to be had from a job well done.

Currently in the US it is imperative for physicians to purchase malpractice insurance to cover them against financial judgements from malpractice claims. Different medical specialties have different risks and so the costs vary from medical specialty and geographic area. An average family practitioner or internist may pay $5,000 to $10,000 per year for coverage. But high-risk specialties such as Obstetrics or neurosurgery usually pay in excess of $100,000 per year for insurance coverage! These costs represent significant "overhead" for the physician and drive the increases in physician fees.

Assuming that we as a nation are heading towards a nationalized health care system it should be noted that substantial changes in malpractice tort laws will be part of that. Although it is difficult to get enough information for a comprehensive comparison of malpractice issues in the USA with western European countries that have a nationalized health insurance system there are some conclusions that can be made. Malpractice insurance premiums in European countries are 3-4 times less than for comparable specialists in the USA. Malpractice claims by plaintiffs are substantially less in Europe. It is rare to have jury trials for malpractice in Europe and most cases are adjudicated either by a judge or by an administrative panel. Some countries have adopted "no fault" compensation models for medical misadventures. If and when the transition happens in the USA to a nationalized health care system, the malpractice tort system will also need to be modified. Certainly if physicians become agents/employees of the government then the citizens of the US will be curtailed in their right to press legal malpractice claims in the courts. The trial lawyers in the USA will not be happy campers when the US adopts a European style national health system.

Paying for It

There was a time in the past few decades when the debate was about whether or not health care was a privilege or a right. If judged to be a privilege, then those who could afford insurance or had the financial means to pay out of pocket for medical care were the beneficiaries and all others were just out of luck. If health care was judged to be a civil right, then it was imperative that public funds be applied to help those who could not get or afford insurance. I think that for all intents and purposes that debate is done and over although a few echoes remain among the most conservative of our society. It seems clear that a compassionate society cannot tolerate having a portion of its citizens unable to receive necessary medical care because of inability to pay. But having settled that question it now comes to the question of who is going to pay the medical bills of our citizens. This is a significant issue since National Health Care Expenditures in 2014 consumed 17.5% of GDP (which ranks #1 in the world) on health care working out to an average of $9523 per capita or $3 trillion dollars. Currently the rate of inflation of health care costs is 6.5% with no end in sight! The inflation rate for health care expenses has been double or more the general inflation rate for the economy and that trend has not shown much real signs of changing. Aggravating the problem is the 75 million "baby boomer" generation who are now entering retirement age—an age that is associated with significantly increased costs per individual for health care related problems. The "millennial" generation that follows next is also 75+ million persons so this increasing expense is not going to go away in a generation. How are we as individuals and as a society going to pay for this?

Private insurance has failed to solve the problem. Everyone who has private or employment provided health insurance is aware of the double-digit percent yearly increases in health care insurance premiums. These increasing premiums have also been associated with steep increases in the out of pocket costs for the individual with higher "co-pays" for accessing doctors and hospitals and with high deductibles now commonly $5000 or more before the insurance starts to pay any health care bills. Previous strategies to try to control health care costs and expenses have included Health Maintenance Organizations (HMO) and Preferred Provider Networks (PPN) as well as increasingly enforced insurance denials of high priced services such as MRIs, etc. through a very tough-minded preauthorization process and restrictive drug formularies that increase patient out of pocket costs with the more expensive medications. This trend has led to the demise of many parochial insurance companies and to the merging of the surviving companies into ever bigger national insurance powerhouses. The trend nationally is towards having only a hand full (5-6) of large national health insurers but I don't know of any commentator that predicts that this trend will reduce the cost of medical care or insurance. To the contrary, it is widely expected that having only a few health care insurance "monopoly's" will result in higher medical costs. The Obama administration filed a legal suit aimed to prevent the merger of several large insurance companies for just this reason. Additionally, private employers have looked to find ways to reduce their health care costs and have modified their work force to as many part time workers as possible in order to avoid the requirement of providing health benefits to their employees. The increasing cost to employers for health care insurance benefits for their employees is a major detriment to US economic growth.

The promise of ObamaCare (the Affordable Care Act) was that the health care exchanges, etc. would result in a sharp reduction in the number of uninsured individuals and would do that at a reduced overall cost because millions of newly insured patients would spread the cost of health care out over many more individuals. It is well documented that ObamaCare failed to deliver on this promise. Although many more previously uninsured individuals have been able to obtain health insurance, the overall number of uninsured individuals has not been significantly reduced. What has happened is that many employers reduced work provided health insurance benefits, many people thus displaced from insurance have not signed up for ObamaCare health insurance plans, those with pre-existing medical conditions that were not previously insured have become insured, healthy young individuals have not embraced the need for health insurance and the costs of delivering care through these insurance plans has increased rather than decreased. The promise that "you can keep your own doctor" and that the average family would reduce their health care premiums $2500 per year just did not materialize. And now, many of the health care insurance companies that offered insurance through the ObamaCare exchanges are withdrawing because they have been losing money by the bucketfulls! When I am in my most cynical mood I think that this was all according to plan—the progressive political movement really wants to move us to a nationalized health care system and needed to show the failure of the private health insurance industry to control costs so as to justify legislation that will move us to a European style national health insurance program. Another eight years of a Democratic-progressive administration should get that job done! Even a Republican administration will have a hard time turning the tide that is inexorably leading us to a crisis of health care financing. It is clear that ObamaCare was only an intermediate solution on the way to a single payer national health care system.

Government health insurance—Medicare and Medicaid—is likewise failing. Medicare expenditures in 2014 were $618.7 billion and Medicaid expenditures were $495.8 billion a combined total of over 1 trillion dollars! These two government funded programs only account for a third or total health care spending, the remainder is through private insurance funded mechanisms. And the 75 million baby boomers are just coming on to the Medicare program, thus severely aggravating the problem for the next 20 years. The inclusion of prescription drug coverage on Medicare during the George W. Bush presidency significantly increased Medicare costs. Medicare and Medicaid represent 25% of the entire Federal budget—the single largest part of the budget. (As a point of comparison Social Security accounts for 24%, Defense 16% and interest on the national debt 6% of the Federal budget.) From the early days of Medicare when physicians and hospitals submitted their bills and Medicare paid them on a "fee for service" cost basis there have been many new Medicare programs to try to reign in the cost to Medicare for insuring the elderly in our country. This started with DRGs as discussed earlier and CPT codes with "Medicare approved amounts" that paid on a Medicare pay schedule and did not pay the doctor or hospitals their billed amount. Medicare now pays 80% of the Medicare "approved" amount of the doctor's fee with the patient responsible for the remaining 20%. Private Medicare supplement insurance was developed and sold to patients to cover the 20%. Medicare HMOs (Medicare Advantage Plans) were also developed putting these patients under the insurance administration of a large private health insurance company with all the usual restrictions and red tape that these arrangements entail. These plans are failing financially as well. Now in the current years Medicare is trying to swing away from a "fee for service" payment—they refer to it as a "pay for performance" system-- with a variety of new rules that are now just being completed and will go into effect in 2017. These are labeled as "pay for quality" programs and include the new MACRA and MIPS regulations as discussed above, as well as "bundling" of the hospital payments to a single global fee that the hospital and the physicians must share, to ACOs where groups of physicians are put at risk with Medicare for managing the costs associated with providing care to the Medicare enrolled patient. To date the current ACO participants have in large part failed to curtail medical costs and some are suggesting that this program has failed already in only its first few years of operation. The end result is that physicians are being put financially at risk for Medicare costs. These new rules include a requirement for the electronic medical record (EMR) with physician reporting requirements to demonstrate "quality" care (all according to Medicare set quality care guidelines) which are associated with the threat—nay the certainty—of payment reductions if the physician does not meet the benchmark "quality" levels. As I have previously stated in this monograph: If Medicare had set out with the overtly expressed purpose of making compliance with Medicare rules and regulations so onerous as to make every physician decide that they would no longer see Medicare patients they couldn't have done it more successfully than they have! Most physicians are not happy with the coming new world of Medicare. Likewise, most physicians are not happy with the corporate controlled private health care insurance industry either. Something has got to change and that change will be a fully nationalized health care system with one payer ("Medicare for all"), one set of rules and administration and full public payment for medical care in the USA. I am not happy about this, but it appears to be inevitable.

So right now, in 2016 physicians are in the worst possible world as far as the business side of medical practice is concerned. Office overhead for practicing medicine is 55% or more with increasing costs ahead to comply with the new world of demonstrating compliance with "quality of care" rules. The metrics that define "quality care" are different from insurance to insurance so the physician must try to comply with multiple lists of rules and regulations. More non-physician staff and more expensive computer hardware and software costs are required to comply thus seriously eroding physician revenues. Health care costs are high—highest in the world per capita; private and government health insurance costs are out of control. The physician is increasingly targeted as the "deep pocket" upon which the financial woes of health care are to be balanced. In an attempt to be more efficient, productive and cost responsible physicians are using digital technology and patients are complaining that "the doctor never looks at me, only at the computer screen!" To get payment from insurance physicians must spend more and more time filling up the EHR—some estimates are that 40% of the physician's time is spent just polishing up the digital records! Is there any wonder that physician burnout is at epidemic proportions! Is it any wonder that new models of medical practice like "direct primary care" that bypasses insurance all together are gaining more and more traction? Why would any fresh-faced young college student want to enter into the profession of medicine with the mess that is the current system? This is the major reason why 80% of newly minted physicians are opting for "employed" status, working usually for a large insurance company who guarantees them some stable income while insulating them from the business management nightmare that is health care in America.

In my opinion, all of the current insurance programs for payment reform and control that I have mentioned will fail. Some have failed already! I think that everyone who studies the issue would need to conclude the same thing. I am sure that all of the "policy wonks" know that these measures will not work and are not sustainable. The progressive political agenda does not see these current Medicare reforms as the end game. It is clear to me that the only solution is to quit tinkering with the current system. The current system is dying if not already dead! A new health care system (by system I mean the business aspect of paying for medical care) is needed. Given the fact that it is absolutely not possible to go back to the original "fee for service" model that was started in the early days of Medicare and private insurance the only solution is to move to a totally nationalized health care system. This has been the progressive political agenda for decades and it is clear that we are on the threshold of realizing that liberal dream. I see it happening in one of two ways: (1) Legislation is passed to move to a single payer insurance system—the so-called "Medicare for all" system. All private insurance ends, government funding (public tax funding) and control of medical expenditures becomes the new model. All physicians, hospitals and other medical care providers become government employees with government imposed salaries, work requirements, and administration by career government administrators. Professional unions bloom. Tort reform must be a necessary part of this to make suing the government for malpractice a very rare thing indeed. Control of medical costs by rationing of medical services—not by denying services but by long waits for specific services: rationing by que! Only time will tell, but I am certain that the quality of experience that the public would have with this system would be a step down from the current system. (2) A graded move into national health insurance with a single payer insurance— "Medicare for all" to cover expenses but the maintenance of private hospitals, physicians, and other health care providers who must look to that single source of payment for medical services. New and very restrictive rules and regulations typical of any government regulating agency would be developed defining the way in which the hospitals and physicians interact with the new scheme. These new rules would be enforced by government sanctions including fines and threats of jail time for the worst offenders since these regulations would have the weight of "law" behind them. Financially enforced compliance with patient care guidelines would be required of the doctors and hospitals. With time, the dissatisfaction within that system would rise to such a level that the physicians and hospitals would all succumb to the pressures and a fully nationalized system like scenario 1 above eventually comes into place.

I don't like the final solution but I am oh so grateful that I will not be a practicing physician during the transition to it. I believe that the new breed of physicians practicing under the new scheme will be fundamentally different in temperament, work ethic, and methodology. Government imposed medical guidelines will dictate the patient-physician interaction. I don't believe that health care providers will fall to the level of personal service that is typical of the DOT employee so often joked about, but I don't see that there will be motivation for the physician to go out of their way to provide the degree of personal compassionate care that has been typical of the profession in the past. I do not look forward to being a patient under that regime. Whether or not a nation as large and diverse as the US can make a success of that new system will take decades to answer, but it is inevitable. Already mature European national health systems are failing as manifest by the rise of private pay health care available to those who can afford it. The progressive ideal of one health care system treating all classes of citizens the same is not likely to reached, and the health care system in 20 years from now is entirely unpredictable.

Selected Patient Care Issues

Alternative and Complimentary health care

There is another whole track of medical care that consumes money in the US—what is called alternative or complementary care. This care consists of vitamins, essential oils, nutritional products, herbal remedies, acupuncture, massage therapy and chiropractic. Current reports peg the amount of money spent on these treatments at about $34 billion per year (about $115 per capita per year.) This is a relatively minimal cost compared to the cost of traditional medical care and represents an amount equal to about 1.5% of the total amount Americans spend on medical care. Americans spend $21 billion per year on herbal and vitamin supplements and $12 billion to $15 billion on chiropractic care, acupuncture and massage therapy. As a component of total health care costs this obviously represents a near negligible amount of money. Some chiropractic care is insurance reimbursed, very little acupuncture is insurance reimbursed and essentially no massage therapy is insurance reimbursed. If these costs were totally illuminated there would be no positive effect on the crisis in health care costs.

If alternative treatments were expanded in the USA could that result in a less expensive method of delivering health care to our population? Well, that depends upon what your end point is. If alternative treatments were effective in the treatment of our most expensive illnesses—cancer, heart disease, chronic lung disease and diabetes and arthritis—then there may be some reason to answer in the affirmative. However, none of the alternative treatment options have been demonstrated to be effective therapy for these illnesses. Adding these treatments and adjunctive therapy to traditional medical care has also not been shown to add significant cost saving therapeutic value either.

In my experience, people who advocate alternative and complimentary therapies do so with the conviction of a zealot...it is a religion with them! They use self-administered herbal and "natural" treatments to treat self-diagnosed illnesses to the exclusion of traditional medical care. It is always an uncomfortable situation for the physician to have family members, or friends or people they meet at social gatherings who are alternative health care zealots. I remember one day that a neighbor of mine who sells and advocated "essential oils" called me about her young son who was ill with a persistent fever, body aches and a cough and told me that she had used several different oils to no avail and the young man was still sick and getting worse. "What would you recommend?" she asked to which I replied as kindly as I could muster "take your son to the doctor!" I also had another neighbor call about an ill family member and told me that she had consulted with a neighbor who was an herbalist, another neighbor who was an essential oil practitioner and now was calling me to see what I thought she should do! Again, my answer was "take your child to the doctor!" My point in these illustrations is that it is likely that many individuals delay diagnosis and appropriate treatment because of their reliance on alternative health care. They do this to their own detriment. I have been unable to find any studies that answer whether or not these individuals end up with more expensive traditional medical care with worse outcomes because of this delay or not, but I suspect that is the case at least now and then. As expensive as "modern medicine" is, it clearly has improved the health and longevity of the general population.   There is no place for the inclusion of alternative and complimentary therapies as a component of a plan to improve the health outcomes of the US population at a reduced cost.

While not strictly on the topic of alternative and complimentary medical treatment the subject of medical quackery needs a little discussion. Fortunately, medical quacks represent a very small percentage of medical practitioners but they are out there in almost every town of any size. The trademark of a medical quack is a practitioner who claims to have some special secret knowledge that is either unknown to the general medical practitioner, or that is actively suppressed by traditional medicine because doctors don't want people to get well since they make money on the care of the sick. Medical quacks may have forged credentials, but by in large they are physicians educated in the usual medical schools and post graduate training programs that seem to go off the rails as soon as they have their medical licenses in hand. They usually depend upon word of mouth advertising or may take out adds in the media advertising their especial cures or treatments. It would be nice if I could say that these practitioners are sincere believers in their cures but since their treatments are usually not covered by insurance, they do a nice cash upon treatment business with low overhead costs. It seems that they are not really medical pioneers but medical privateers! It would be nice if I could say that they are harmless and only separate gullible people from their money, but their treatments often do harm if for no other reason than delaying the provision of proven medical treatments. It is mysterious why some patients seem to get symptom relief from their treatments, but I believe it is because of a variation of the "placebo effect" that has been repeatedly demonstrated to produce a positive response in about 40% of persons. I had an old high school classmate who developed generalized seizures after graduation and was on prescription medication which controlled the seizures. However, he decided to go to an alternative practitioner and after a series of treatments was told that "you can stop taking your medication now, you are cured!" He took their advice and subsequently ended up in the emergency room with uncontrollable seizures that resulted in multiple bone and spinal fractures before the seizures could be stopped. Medical quackery is not harmless. There is certainly no place in the national discussion for inclusion of these practitioners in a comprehensive medical treatment system.

The Secrets of a Long and Healthy Life

I am often asked by family, friends or at social gatherings what I think are the keys to living a long and healthy life. My usual answer is this: There are 3 secrets to a long and healthy life; good genes, good habits, and good luck! Nowhere in that formula is mentioned good doctor, good hospital, good insurance, or a nationalized health care system! That is because the health care system—medical science, doctors, etc.—is about repairing people who have developed health care problems, but is not about preventing those problems.

Also, it could be successfully argued that the health and welfare of the American public has been most improved by the modern application of the application of clean water sources and modern sewage disposal and treatment. Doctors may be able to rescue your good health, but having good health is for now out of their hands. Some would say that doctors should promote good health practices by their patients. How could anyone disagree with that? But the fact is, that doctors cannot make their patients do what is best for their health. Public awareness campaigns and school based educational teaching can be effective in promoting healthy life styles, but in the end individual people must take hold of the responsibility of being as healthy as they can be.

There is no question that genetics plays a powerful role in health and wellness. Most of the major diseases in our modern society have strong genetic predispositions including cancer, heart disease, and diabetes and even obesity. Now that the human genome has been worked out, there is becoming more and more evidence of the power of genetics in both health and disease. The coming decade promises to be exciting for medical science as we progress from understanding the human genome to being able to manipulate it for therapeutic advantage. The message of genetics to you as an individual is this: if there is a strong history of a certain disease in your family line you should take whatever measures are available, including life-style changes and medications or other medical therapies to try to delay as long as possible what your genes have in store for you. Also, with the increasing understanding of genetics as it relates to disease, expect that there will be measures taken to categorize you into risk pools and that government or insurance policies may be developed that may treat you differently based upon your genetic risks. It is clear that some genetic groups will have increased risks of serious and expensive diseases and there will at least be debate about whether or not these groups should be treated differently from the general population insofar as paying for treatment is concerned. Additionally, it is becoming clear that certain genetic "types" respond better or worse to medical treatments and it will become increasingly possible to tailor medical treatments to the ones that will work best for your genetic type. I know that this sounds like the stuff that dystopian novels and movies are made of but it is clear that the reality of our increasing knowledge of genetics as it relates to disease will have potential ramifications in policy decisions about medical issues as we enter this "brave new world." The technology to quickly and accurately do DNA testing at an affordable price may lead to requirements for DNA testing as medical policy makers try to manage medical care costs and discriminate on the basis of medical science what treatments may be offered to what patients. The societal discussion of these issues, and many others that have genetic attributes (such as temperament, leadership qualities, intelligence, aptitude, physical characteristics, etc.) is just beginning and it no longer is in the realm of science fiction! A whole new set of rules about personal privacy will need to be crafted to protect your genetic information from misuse and abuse. Measures to protect you from discrimination because of your genetic risks will need to be crafted. But on balance, I believe that we may be on the verge of exciting medical breakthroughs as the medical science aspects of the human genome mature.

Good habits cannot be over emphasized. A story is told about a geriatrician who is researching the secret to a long life. He decides to go to Florida where a lot of people retire and find some old folks to study. He comes upon three old guys on a bench overlooking a beach and decides to start with them. "Can you tell me to what you attribute your long life" the researcher asks the first fellow. "Well, I grew up on a farm in the country. We did hard work. We grew most of our own food. We got up early and went to bed early. There was lots of fresh air and exercise." "Very interesting" said the researcher "how old are you?" "Eighty-five" was the reply. He then moved to the second fellow and asked the same question to which the man answered "Well, I grew up in the city. We knew that there was pollution and unhealthy stuff that we were exposed to so we didn't smoke, or drink alcohol. We took lots of vitamins and we went to the gym to exercise." "How old are you, sir?" the researcher asked. "Eighty-one was his reply." Thinking he was seeing a pattern here the researcher moved to the last old man asking again the same question. He replied "Well, I was not like these other fellows at all. I smoked, drank heavily, chased women, stayed up late, never exercised and I ate mostly at fast food joints." In surprise, the researcher asked "so how old are you?" The third man replied "I'm 39!" Of course, this is just a story to illustrate the point that our life style choices have a great deal of effect upon or health and longevity. It is now universally accepted that smoking is the foremost preventable cause of cancer and heart disease. Alcohol likewise is associated with many adverse health conditions. Obesity is an epidemic in our society. Lack of exercise is a killer. Stressful jobs and environments can shorten our lives and make us sick. Those among us who fail to avoid these preventable causes of excessive and early morbidity and mortality make up a disproportionate percentage of those upon whom the medical profession spends time and money trying to treat, cure and rehabilitate. Now, we could enter into a discussion about whether or not those people who do not follow good health practices should pay extra into the insurance scheme to compensate for their increase expenses due to their life style choices, but that is a policy debate that is above my pay grade. But I must point out that you do not have any control over what genes you inherited, and the discussion in the next paragraph will be about "good luck" that is not under our control, so it seems prudent to do what you have the power to do to make yourself as healthy as you can be. It is socially irresponsible for any individual to expect the rest of us to pay for their poor choices when they have the ability to choose differently!

Good luck! We use that phrase all the time when we interact with others. But who can control random chance? As the saying goes: "Shit happens" and there is little that can be done to prevent it. Worse than that, people can just be in the wrong place at the wrong time. But in some respects we make our own luck. It has been said that the most common "last words" of a Redneck are "Hey you-all, watch this!" Taking foolish and unwise chances hoping against the odds that things will work out well for us invites bad luck. So, put on your seat belts when you drive your car. Put on your helmets when you ride you bike, and don't buy that Harley Davidson that you have had your eye on for years. Don't take illegal narcotics, or any narcotics for that matter other than for very short-term pain relief. Be careful with sharp objects. Look out where you step. Avoid dark alleys at night in big cities. Of course, the medical profession will try their best to rescue you from your mishaps, but avoiding the mishaps in the first place is your responsibility.

I grew up in the 1960s and a common personal motto then was: "Live hard, die young and leave a good-looking corpse!" Given the fact that the major driver of increasing health care costs is the chronic diseases of the aging population maybe we should promote such a life style? Of course, I am not serious about that thought! The average life expectancy in the US now 78.8 years and has been steadily rising over the last 5 decades. Most adults will develop some type of chronic disease that will consume medical resources to treat. The average adult age 60 is on 2.2 medications daily. We have made great strides in helping people live longer and better. But, the burden of chronic disease in the USA is heavy and the cost of dealing with it is extreme. If as I predict we will shortly enter into a publicly financed nationalized health care system it is a matter of personal responsibility to do all that you can do to reduce your own personal cost to the system. When a nationally financed system is in place expect there to be incentives for good health habits and good safety habits and penalties for not doing what is prudent.

Anderson's Curve

Medical science has done wonders...even miracles! Diseases that once had 100% mortality rates are now being successfully treated and sometimes cured. Life expectancy is steadily increasing, and mortality rates from all causes are declining. But that said, we are all still mortal and sometime we will die. Medical science can extend life but it cannot prevent death. And there comes a time in each individual's life that they usually transition from fully functional and independent to minimally functional and dependent. Of course some people die suddenly in their prime—an accident, homicide, a fatal acute heart attack, etc. changes this scenario for them from one of gradual decline from independence to dependency to acute demise. But that is not what I am talking about here. In the normal situation, we continue to grow stronger, bigger and better until about age 26 or 28 and then the body crests the optimal health curve and starts the long decline towards old age and deterioration. This deterioration affects every organ system in predictable ways. The hair thins, the skin wrinkles, the muscles lose mass and strength, the balance gets worse, the reflexes slow, the mind processes less efficiently, the skeleton loses bone density, the endurance wanes…. you get the picture! Adding to this curve and steepening the slope of decline is the burden of chronic disease…arthritis, hardening of the arteries, diabetes, hypertension, chronic lung disease, cancer, etc. Some treatments for diseases save your life in the short run but cause a steepening of the curve as a side effect. Then you can add to that burden the superimposition of self-induced factors that steepen the curve such as smoking, alcohol, obesity, physical inactivity and poor protein calorie nutrition. Every individual's curve on this chart is different in slope, but the pattern is the same for everyone.

When I was a hospitalist at the LTAC for the last 8 years of my career the patients I cared for had all come to me from another hospital where they had been acutely hospitalized for a medical or surgical problem. They all had complications that required them to have a prolonged hospital stay. Commonly these patients were old with multiple chronic medical problems. Many were severely debilitated and were bed bound or required a lot of assistance to get in and out of bed and do any self-care. They were dependent. I often had to try to explain to them and their families why they had digressed from being independent at home before their illness to fully dependent after their illness. Many times, family members would say "I just don't understand it, he was doing so well before all of this happened." Almost always on closer questioning it was apparent that the patient had been in declining health before the medical event becoming frailer and less energetic but because they could take care of their own bathing, toileting, clothing and feeding they and family members felt they were doing "OK". I explained to them that in the face of a declining overall health as described above an acute event—such as a medical or surgical illness—can overwhelm their bodies capacity to compensate and acute dependency is the result. I also explained that because of their declining overall health, this acute event would be very difficult to recover from and that it was very unlikely that the patient would be able to recover back to the level of independence they had before the acute illness. The nurses and case managers at the LTAC came to describe this discussion as "Anderson's Curve". The concept was clearly not original with me, but the principles were easily understood and most patients and their families were able to grasp a hold of the fact that what was before was not going to be the situation after the medical catastrophe. Extreme effort on the part of the patient with attention to excellent nutrition, physical and occupational therapy and a lot of time would be required to see improvement from dependency to independence with no guarantee that persistent dependency would not be the outcome.

In this country, we seem to be very reluctant to face up to the fact that life comes to an end. We tend to think that one more treatment, one more surgery, one more new medication will restore us to our former health and vigor. Vitamins and "nutraceuticals" are bought and consumed in a hope for a return to our earlier state of health and vigor. Anderson's curve is not generally acknowledged by patients or by their doctors. Oncologists seem to always offer one more round of treatment. Surgeons seem to offer hope with some new surgical technique. Physicians make adjustments to or add a new medicine that is supposed to turn the tide of illness in a positive direction. But there is no cure for mortality! Getting old is not for sissies! False hope is engendered in the patient and their family. The treatments recommended are offered in a futile effort to stave off dependency and death for a little more time. Many times the added treatment causes suffering and may even shorten life due to side effects. Cancer patients with no chance for a cure want to continue "fighting" as if it is morally wrong to admit that the illness will win and that if we fail to struggle against that eventuality we are somehow "quitters"—and nobody wants to be known as a quitter! For some reason both physicians and patients are reluctant to turn the conversation over to managing the end of life. Discussions of end of life care are always awkward, and frequently contentious when multiple family members view the goals of treatment differently. Patients often hear "what they want to hear" rather than what their physicians actually said about their prognosis and their options for care. This too often leads to the end of life being spent in hospitals, LTACs, care centers, etc. suffering through invasive and uncomfortable medical treatments. Rather than "dying with dignity" too many of us die in hospital beds, tied to ventilators and dialysis machines and high tech medical treatments that will not return us to functional independent life. Hospice care is rejected as "giving up" when in fact hospice care can make the end of life more comfortable and in some cases may extend life beyond what might happen if aggressive treatments with potential side effects are administered. Recently published (jamainternalmedicine.com 8/1/2016) was a survey done among a group of patients aged 60+ all of whom had end stage "terminal" illnesses ranging from cancer to heart and lung disease. In that survey they were asked to rank some issues compared to death—were these things worse than, equal to or better than death. Six things were ranked worse than or equivalent with death: (in rank order 1-6) lack of bowel and bladder control; needing to rely on a ventilator to live; inability to get out of bed; being confused all the time; needing to rely on a feeding tube to live; and needing to have constant care provided for them. It is obvious that patients are able to judge what things make life worth living and what things are worse than continuing living. What we need is a safe forum where these issues can be discussed not only between physicians and patients but between the greater public as well.

    There is another side to this as well. The cost of continuing aggressive medical care when it is not going to prolong life or the quality of life is immense. 30% of Medicare spending is on patients in their last one year of life. 40% of that amount is spent in the last one month of life... a number that is approaching $100 billion per year. If we as a nation are serious about reducing health care spending, and if we want to "bend the curve" of the yearly increases in Medicare costs our best opportunity is in addressing the cost of futile medical care at the end of life. No other proposed program—not MACRA, MIPS, ACOs or bundled Medicare payments has anywhere near the savings opportunity as does a serious discussion about the expense of end of life aggressive medical treatments. A great fear expressed about ObamaCare was that there would be "death panels" to decide who got treatments and who didn't. This fear was couched in terms of unfair preference given to some people but withheld from others. The idea that denying medical treatments to anyone who wants them is immoral just has to be put aside in the national conversation! We now have enough experience and data dealing with medical issues that we can predict accurately which patients are on a trajectory to death and will not benefit from the application of aggressive medical treatment. In my estimation, it is immoral to apply futile treatments to those people. End of life care such as is delivered with Hospice and other similar programs allows the patient to acknowledge their coming demise, removes from them false hope, helps them make choices about what things are the most important to them as they face their own mortality, and allows the family to become settled with the concept that life is not forever. We will soon enter an era of universal government health insurance where everyone has access to medical services, but until we embrace the fact that no one lives forever and that the end of life is a stage that can be managed with dignity we will not be a compassionate society! The proper management of end of life health care is essential to the patient's interests as well as to the national financial interests.

    We must address the question of medical futility in order to progress into the next era of medical care. No longer is the question asked of medical technology "can we do it" since medical science continues to prove that "yes we can". The bigger question is "should we do it"? At what point does continued application of medical therapy to an individual reach a point of diminishing returns such that further treatment is futile? Does the extension of life by a few months in a terminal cancer patient by another round of chemotherapy, surgery or radiotherapy represent a positive value to us? Does offering kidney dialysis to an octogenarian make medical and ethical sense? Does replacing a failing heart valve in a 90-year-old represent a positive value? Is the mission statement for medical care to extend life to the last possible day regardless of cost in terms of financial resources and patient suffering? I have had many conversations with patient's families when their loved one was in a coma, on life support with maximal medications and no signs that recovery was going to happen. Many times the family has said in essence: "we don't want to be responsible for the decision to let dad die, we want God to take him if it is his time." Their decision was to press on with active medical care against all hope. As sympathetic as I am with that desire to not feel the weight of guilt for the decision to "turn off the machines" I have to respond to the families as kindly as I can that "if God was in charge, your dad would already be gone. It is only because we have interfered with God that he is still alive." In our secular world that concept is a little harder to state, but the point is that there comes a time when further medical care is futile. There even becomes a time when further medical care is unkind to the patient. Allowing the patient or the family to choose whether or not to apply medical technology when the cost/benefit analysis is unfavorable is putting off the medical profession's responsibility onto the shoulders of people who have no experience or expertise in making an informed decision. Since medical resources are finite and expensive we need to address as a society when it is no longer acceptable to continue to add on more treatment when the return in length of life and independent functionality is minimal or absent. Of course, in making such hard decisions there will be cases pointed to of when a decision to treat was made and the patient had a miraculous recovery to independence, but it must also be acknowledged that these cases are exceptionally rare. No one gets out of this world alive. Can we as a society afford the financial and emotional cost of unlimited expenditure of resources to obtain the very last day of life possible for every individual? Expect that to be a hot topic for debate when a nationalized health care program is fully mature.

"But" you might say "it isn't right to do nothing just because the patient has no chance to be cured or given a significant length of life by applying some medical or surgical treatment!" That mental frame of mind is based in the concept that to do something is better than doing nothing, and that we have to "fight" the battle against death even though it is clear that we cannot win. However, not giving another round of chemotherapy, or doing another surgery, or not putting the patient on life support machines, or applying some other treatment is not the same as doing nothing. Once we can get away from this type of thinking it is apparent that there is a whole arsenal of things that we can actively do for the patient who is faced with a terminal, incurable and fatal illness. First, we can relieve them and their loved ones from the burden of unreasonable hope that clouds their thinking and keeps them from facing the inevitable. Next, we can honestly talk to the patient and family and give them a clear picture of how things are likely to proceed and give them a scientifically supported time line to base decisions upon. These two things can give the patient and their family mental clarity that will be a blessing to them as they proceed through the terminal weeks or months. (Studies have shown that in oncology practice even when the oncologist feels they have given an objective statement of how poor the prognosis is even with therapy the patients and their families seem only to hear the part about some other therapy that could be "tried" thinking that it will make some significant difference in the outcome. The patient seems to not hear the part that nothing will make a significant difference and then may opt to try one more round of chemotherapy, etc.) Then we can help with symptom control for pain, nausea, weakness, shortness of breath, etc. that will allow the patient to be as awake, conscious and comfortable as possible through the end game. We can assist the patient and their family in making final arrangement plans so that they are not left to the few days following the patient's demise when grieving is at its most intense. And, most importantly, we can allow the patient to decide what is most important to them in these final stages of their life and try to make those things happen. These things constitute a whole universal of things that "can be done" even when there is no possibility of a cure or a long disease-free interlude. These things are "low tech" but highly effective and have been shown to increase patient's satisfaction with the care provided and in some cases has a better effect on life duration than active medical treatments.

Medical Uncertainty

In medical school the student is taught the process of differential diagnosis. This is the process where the student assembles all of the available symptoms reported by the patient, couples those with findings on physical examination and lab and X-ray reports and then goes through the process of mentally making a prioritized list of the possible diagnoses that could account for the situation. This is important because the self-same symptoms can be seen in many different disorders. For instance, a patient may complain of chest pain and think they are having a heart attack, but chest pain may be due to chest wall inflammation, heart disease, pulmonary embolism, esophageal ulcer, esophageal spasm, anxiety attack, trauma, or several other causes nowhere near as serious as a heart attack.

Other considerations that the doctor needs to consider are the age and sex of the patient, the patient's family history of diseases, other associated symptoms such as heartburn or shortness of breath, and findings on examination of the chest and heart of the patient. When the situation is not clear after a good interview, and by physical examination then the physician needs to consider how they might narrow down the possibilities by either further testing or sometimes a therapeutic trial of treatment for what seems the most likely diagnosis. Throughout this process the doctor mentally constructs a prioritized list of the most likely diagnosis and when they are adequately certain of the diagnosis a treatment program is suggested. An old adage we are taught in medical school is "when you hear hoof beats don't think zebras!" This means that common diseases are the most likely cause— "common diseases occur commonly"—and rare diseases should not be on the top of your differential diagnosis list. Now, it is true that rare diseases do occur but again "rare diseases occur rarely". The art of medical science is to sift through the symptoms and signs and lab and X-ray reports and discover whether you are dealing with a horse or a zebra. Patients are notoriously poor at this process and in our age of media hype and internet they often decide that they have whatever the "disease of the month" is that is all over the media. Treating a person as if they have a heart attack when what they have is an inflamed rib joint with the sternum is a waste of time, money and emotional capital. On the other hand, treating a patient who is having a heart attack as though they have esophageal reflux is dangerous for the patient's well-being and even for their life.

    Admittedly some doctors are too quick to make a diagnosis and end up treating the patient for the wrong diagnosis. There is a fine line sometimes between trying to be quick and efficient in making a diagnosis and starting treatment and taking too long to exhaust all the possibilities before trying to treat the problem. Acid blockers don't treat heart attacks and chest wall pain does not need to lead to a coronary angiogram. The doctor's experience and depth of knowledge is key in finding the right balance. In this regard, it is my opinion that "specialists" are not the best doctors to formulate and pursue the differential diagnosis. For instance, if you have chest pain you should not go to a cardiologist because if the chest pain is not your heart the cardiologist will just tell you that "it's not your heart" and tell you to go back to your primary care doctor. There is another adage in medicine: "If your only tool is a hammer the whole world looks like a nail!" Sometimes a specialist will spend your time and money doing all the tests that are in their "tool bag" without really taking the time to do an initial assessment of whether or not your symptom really is in their scope of specialty. This wastes your time and costs money that is essentially wasted. On the other hand, the primary care doctor who does not have adequate experience or depth of knowledge will not be able to formulate an appropriate differential diagnosis so they may send you to one specialist after another wasting time and money as well and trying your patience while you await a proper diagnosis and treatment.

Another aspect of this is that most diseases present themselves in the usual "textbook" manner and so the most obvious diagnosis is the right diagnosis most of the time. But some problems present themselves in atypical ways. For instance, it is well known that heart attack in women often presents with symptoms other than chest pain—such as nausea or lightheadedness-- so the experienced doctor must be aware that the usual symptoms may not be present even for the most common of diseases. Sometimes it is prudent in formulating a differential diagnosis to list the most serious or life threating disease at the top of the doctor's list even if the symptoms and signs are not typical since the worst possible scenario is to miss treating a life-threatening diagnosis because it was not considered in the appropriate time frame.

Now in the midst of all of the uncertainty that exists in the practice of medicine even the best doctor will miss the right diagnosis now and then or treat a patient for a problem they do not have. I remember seeing a cartoon once with a physician looking at a patient who was sitting on an examination table: "Doctor, I hope you can treat what I have" the patient said to which the doctor replied "Lady I hope you have what I can treat!" The doctor will need to remain on his guard about the diagnosis until it is clear that the treatment prescribed is solving the problem. The most common causes of symptoms not resolving as expected are: (1) The patient did not comply with the treatment as prescribed—this is way more common than most people may realize and if not considered by the doctor it will lead to multiple different attempts to treat the problem with different medications or treatments, each one failing in turn because of patient non-compliance. A corollary of this problem is when the patient is not only non-compliant with the prescribed treatment but is actively doing things that interfere with the treatment such as continuing to drink alcohol when they are being treated for alcoholic liver disease, or continuing to eat a high salt diet while being treated for high blood pressure, or eating ice cream while being treated for diabetes. (2) The diagnosis is wrong and a different diagnosis needs to be considered. The patient needs to have trust in the doctor's desire to solve their problem, and needs to comply with prescribed treatments. And the patient needs to stick with the doctor through the process rather than flitting from one doctor to the next because treatments don't work immediately. At the same time the doctor needs to do whatever is necessary to be sure that the proper diagnosis is established. It is my opinion that it is better to spend the money and time up front to do what it takes to make a proper diagnosis than to make a quick diagnosis that is wrong. The biggest expense in medical care is not the cost of proper treatment, but the cost of incorrect diagnosis with the prescription of the wrong treatment.

Now, I have spent a lot of time in previous chapters discussing the new model of medical care that is evolving over the last decade and will eventually conclude in a national health care system with government funded health insurance. A big part of that is the EHR (electronic medical record) and the "pay for quality" transition. One pitfall in this transition is concerning this very topic of medical uncertainty. In the coming system the doctor will be required to demonstrate by his EHR notes that they are compliant with federally mandated treatment guidelines. It will be imperative that the doctor show that all of the "boxes" are checked according to the one size fits all guidelines for every patient diagnosis. If the doctor fails to do that they either won't get paid or will get paid a discounted fee, or even penalized financially and pay what amounts to a fine for non-compliance with the quality guidelines. The doctor's incentive will be to treat you for what the guideline requires rather than to tailor your treatment to your particular unique and personal diagnosis. This will start with the most common diagnoses like diabetes, heart disease, cancer etc. but as the system matures it will be comprehensive for all medical problems. It will be more important to the system that the doctor treats you according to guidelines for what they say you have than to actually make the proper diagnosis. Those patients with uncertain diagnoses will be forced into "boxes" on an electronic ledger sheet for which they do not have a definite "fit". Patients will find themselves subjected to treatment protocols that don't really solve their problems. This is in contrast to the emerging field of genetic medicine that holds promise for tailoring treatments to the patient based upon their unique genetics. Treatment guidelines are not by themselves a problem, but when they are coupled with a highly bureaucratic payment system that demands uniformity of reporting there is high likelihood of undesirable outcomes. What derives from the guidelines is a specific list of required actions that the doctor must take and document whether or not it helps resolve the patient's symptoms. In its most extreme form this bureaucratic approach to medical treatment will not only be frustrating to the patient and the physician but may lead to patient harm as "square pegs" are forced into "round" holes. One thing is for sure: the bureaucratic formulation of the treatment guidelines will always lag behind the advances in medical care. In that lag time patients will be harmed because of insurance mandated policies. Physicians are already up in arms about imposed treatment guidelines and excessive documentation requirements…don't expect that problem to get better as the new system of health care matures. I will say it again: if Medicare had set out with the express purpose of formulating policies that would make physicians want to stop seeing Medicare patients they could not have done a better job of it! This is what happens when you allow non-physician politicians and bureaucrats to design a medical care system.

Snake Oil

There have always been snake-oil salesmen prowling the edges of traditional medical care offering secret formulas and cures with promises of miraculous results. In our modern era these cures take out full page advertisements in magazines and newspapers with a targeted population of potential customers. Now in more recent years the internet has become a prime source of sensational claims about herbs, vitamins, mechanical devices (especially anything that works with a "laser") and treatments all promising results "or your money back"! And popular TV talk-shows also spend whole segments on promoting some new cure. They also popularize rare diseases making it appear as though there is an epidemic of ill health and describing symptoms that are so common that every viewer is convinced that they have the "disease of the month". Some of the currently popular diseases of the month are gluten sensitive enteropathy (celiac disease—this disease has actually declined in frequency but the number of people on gluten free diets has increased substantially in the last few years), "leaky bowel syndrome", Hashimoto's disease, and abnormal methylation disorder. Always popular is fibromyalgia and chronic fatigue but often these disorders are repackaged to make them appeal to a larger population base. Lyme disease seems to be surging in the last decade as well. Miracle cures are so common for obesity that it is almost comical. Essential oils are a multibillion dollar per year industry. There are always new secretly formulated vitamin combinations that will fix anything from athlete's foot to bad breath! Juices extracted from exotic fruits have always been popular and every few years some "scientist" seems to walk out of the jungle having discovered a new exotic fruit that contains the elixir of life and health.

    A common thread through all of these iterations on the old snake oil theme is that they come and go in fairly short cycles and often are seen to resurface slightly repackaged a few years later. I think what happens is they each take their turn saturating the market and as the appeal of one version of snake oil wanes another rises to take its place. This is true also of the disease of the month. Usually the disease of the month has so many symptoms that are not specific that everyone will have to wonder if they have them. Symptoms such as fatigue, mental fogginess, muscle aches and pains, diffuse abdominal discomforts, insomnia, weight gain, headaches and back pains are the staples of these diagnoses. Along with that are usually comments about how doctors don't know how to diagnose and treat these diseases and how some practitioner or another has discovered a cure that is being withheld from the public by the greedy medical profession who don't want people to get better because it would hurt their business! Like the snake oil cures these same vague and non-specific symptoms are repackaged from time to time into the new disease of the month. All of this preys on the gullible public who do have many of the symptoms described but do not have the experience or training to be able to discriminate quackery from legitimate medicine. In 2015 alone Americans spent $21 billion dollars on vitamins and herbal supplements that have no demonstrated benefits, and untold billions on other current versions of snake oil. Most of this money is wasted resource since the patient usually finds no real benefit. But, what the heck it was worth a try!

There has clearly been a failure of the medical care system to address the underlying needs of individuals that has kept the snake oil salesmen in business. Some of it is because the big money for medical research is being spent for the study of the biggest issues in medicine: Heart disease and cancer. Cancer research spends about $5 billion per year much of which comes from government grants from the National Institutes of Health. Heart disease research spends over $3 billion per year. The National Institutes of Health spends about $32 billion yearly for medical research and a total of just under $100 billion total is spent by public and private concerns in funding medical research yearly. Pharmaceutical research is a big spender and with big returns if a new miracle drug is discovered, especially if it treats one of the common diseases that effects millions of people. Even if a new drug that is just a variation on an already available drug is developed it can bring large revenues to the pharmaceutical company. Research into the cause of fatigue, insomnia, mental clouding, diffuse aches and pains is essentially nil! In many if not most patients with these complaints lifestyle issues are the root cause but fixing lifestyle habits is a hard business to be in. It is true that heart disease and cancer are the big killers in the USA, but some of the most common reasons that patients go to see their doctors are for the very symptoms that the snake oil salesmen push their wares. If we are going to be able to reduce the cost of providing medical care we must address more aggressively ways to address these common but vague and nonspecific symptoms that keep patients going back to their physicians for help and often turn to the snake oil salesman for relief.

Why does it cost so much?

Health care is big business. In recent years health care costs have approached $3 trillion per year and consumed 17% (1/6th) of the Gross National Product. The United States outranks every other country in the percent of GDP that involves health care. Health Care inflation has routinely been double or more the rate of inflation in general goods and services. Some sectors of the health care industry are extremely profitable: as a sector health care has a profit margin of 15.4%; pharmaceuticals have a profit margin of 20.8%; medical instruments have a 12.5% profit margin; durable medical goods have a 9.5% profit margin. Other sectors of health care have more modest profits: hospitals 3.7% (of course they are paying the high costs of pharmaceuticals, instruments, medical technologies); health insurance plans 3.2%. As a sector of the job market health care jobs as a group are among the highest paying occupations. And, 60% of the health care job growth is in administrative positions that do not have any patient clinical contact thus adding significant expense without any benefit to the patient! The only other endeavor that is so top heavy (administrative) in its employees is government—and we think that nationalizing our health care system will lead to a decrease in cost? A snowball's chance in hell!

Costs for specific disease treatments—surgery and medications-- are in general much higher in the United States than in other countries. As an example, the average price of cardiac bypass surgery in the US is $75,345 which is $30,000 higher than the next highest country; MRI and CT scan are the most expensive of any other country; pharmaceutical prices in the US are about twice the price of Canada, the United Kingdom and Australia. Some have attributed these higher costs to the failure of hospitals and health care providers to negotiate better price contracts with medical vendors. How about price gouging by vendors? On the other hand, Americans have fewer hospital admissions, and fewer doctor visits than the average country. But at the same time Americans must pay more out of pocket in copays and deductibles--$3,442 per capita which is five times more than the next highest spending country. Some attribute the increase medical costs in the US to an oversupply of doctors, especially specialists. But the US has 2.6 physicians per 1000 population compared to Norway which has 4.3, and to the median of 3.2 over a range of 10 countries. Some may say that hospitals drive up the cost of medical care and there are too many hospitals competing for patients to fill their beds, but hospital use in the US is 129 per thousand population compared to a high of 252 in Germany and an average of 164 over a 10-country comparison. Americans are the top consumers of prescription drugs at an average of 2.2 pills per capita. Americans consume more high-tech imaging with MRI scans and PET scans than any other country other than Japan. Americans seem to have a higher rate of chronic disease with 68% of citizens over 65 years old having at least two chronic diseases compared to 56% in Canada and 33% in the United Kingdom. (Data from the Commonwealth Fund, U.S. Health Care from a Global Perspective, October 8, 2015) Other western countries spend on average about half (health care as a % of GDP) as much as the United States on health care. And compared to the cost many metrics of health are lower in the United States than in comparable western wealthy countries. The US ranks last overall compared to 10 wealthy countries in three key measures of health: mortality amenable to medical care; infant mortality; and healthy life expectancy at age 60. (Data from the Commonwealth Fund, *Mirror Mirror on the Wall*, 2014 Update, June 16, 2014)

    As you know, these cost data are at the base of the major debate going on in the country for the last 2 decades: the reformation of health care in the US. At this time in history the US is the only wealthy nation that does not have a nationalized health care system. Many voices are contending that we can make a major difference in both the cost of medical care and the health of the nation by going to a nationalized health system. Countering that argument is that our nation is so large and so diverse that the expectation that installing a western European or Canadian style national health care system in the US is not going to solve the problem. Our national culture favors "fee market" solutions to economic problems—including the price of health care—but it is clear that there is something different about US health care that prevents the free market from working. Unfortunately, our country has a culture of multiplying bureaucrats to administer government programs (Federal plus State government spending accounts for 29% of GDP in the US according to usgovernmentspending.com) The high cost of surgeries, pharmaceuticals, medical equipment and technology in the US suggests that the free market system has failed to provide the economies that would have been and should have been expected. It could be contended that US citizens see their doctor less often and thus put off treatment of their medical conditions until they have progressed to the most expensive to treat stages of disease. Surely this is part of the problem especially for those citizens who are not insured. Additionally, the uninsured in America tend to seek medical care at the most expensive venues, the emergency rooms of hospitals were federal laws prevent the facility from refusing care due to inability to pay. Americans make lifestyle choices at a high rate that have severe health care consequences: overeating that leads to obesity and subsequently higher rates of cardiac disease and diabetes, physical inactivity, drug and alcohol use among the leading culprits. What is clear here is that the health care system in the United States is dysfunctional and because of that it is overly expensive. In fact, we do not really have a health care "system" in the United States. What we have is a profusion of health care systems ranging from private to government funded and comprised of multiple business entities all pursuing their individual interests but all subjected to a set of Federal health care regulations that is ever increasing and impossible to comply with. Powerful lobbies exist (insurance companies, pharmaceutical companies, and hospital companies) spending billions to try to influence federal rules to their advantage. Federal legislation has been piece meal and lacking in an overall plan for guidance in setting public policy. Each new piece of health care legislation—which is politically motivated and caters to specific interests-- seems to result in unintended consequences that results in increased costs—Medicare part "D" and ObamaCare as two recent and prime examples. As I said earlier in this book about it being the worst time to be a physician in the United States, it is likewise the worst time to be a health care business in the United States. Some segments of the health care system are reaping remarkable profits (pharmaceuticals, medical equipment, and durable medical supplies as three prime examples) while others struggle to keep their doors open and see declining incomes and increasing overhead as a result of -federally mandated rules and regulations. Physicians are burned-out, medical clinics are becoming top heavy with administrative and business office personnel, smaller parochial insurance companies are going bankrupt or are being acquired by large national insurance powerhouses, red tape is proliferating at a geometric rate, and the American public is being squeezed by increased out of pocket health care costs. Something has got to give! All of the current measures with Medicare reforms, movement to MACRA, MIPS, ACOs, bundled payment programs is not going to make the problem better. Although I have no confidence that the Federal government can manage anything cost effectively I see no reasonable alternative but to proceed to the next logical step in the nation's progressive journey—a unified national health care system. We can only hope that it is crafted by people who are not pursuing their own self-interest or political agenda and are fully cognizant of the multiple interconnected pieces of health care as a business.

Retirement

    So, the time came for me to retire. I was 65, but still had enough energy and expertise to continue to be a competent physician for a number of years into the future. I felt that I was still at the top of my game, and several of the consulting physicians that I worked with at the LTAC, who were younger than I, still complemented me on the quality of medical care that I provided to my patients. The administrators of the LTAC were receiving very good service from me by their own statements, and I was serving well as the medical director of the LTAC. I did not have to retire due to illness, creeping incompetence, or pressure to step down from patients, hospitals, or colleagues. Practicing medicine was still fulfilling to my personal needs and ego. So, why did I retire? That is a complex answer! I suppose that it was the accumulated effects of the fatigue caused by the demands of medical practice, coupled with a desire to have time to pursue some other items on my "bucket list", added to the fact that I had been fortunate in my personal financial planning and had a very adequate retirement income set up. But, truth be told, I think the real reason was that I was becoming less and less tolerant of the changing landscape of medical care as I have described it in the preceding chapters. Even in my LTAC setting of providing patient medical care, the government and private insurance constraints and restraints were becoming an increasing irritation to me. I did not like what I envisioned was the coming future of medical care. Maybe it was just the "you can't teach old dogs new tricks" part of me, but I could not see that a joyful continuance of medical practice would grace my coming years. It was time to step down from my profession and pursue other interests.

    I found out that I had a hard time letting go of medicine. The science and art of medical care still was important to me. I continued to keep my medical licenses current, but I had to drop my hospital privileges. I continued to keep up with developments in medicine generally, and in my specialty in particular. After spending two-thirds of my life in the practice of medicine, it was part of me. I hoped that I might find some way to contribute my experience and knowledge without having to subject myself to the rigors of medical practice. I applied for and accepted an assignment as a medical advisor to my church's missionary department taking on the task of advising the mission presidents about the health care needs of the young full-time missionaries. This was a full-time service mission without compensation and took me to reside in California for 18 months. I found that the California way of practicing medicine was even more dysfunctional than what I had experienced in Utah. After 18 months, I was ready to be done with this assignment. I investigated doing medical case review for insurance companies, but decided that I had no need financially to work for wages, and besides I had railed against the decisions of insurance companies regarding my patients for many years and just couldn't stomach the idea of being the one who denied medical services to sick patients. Telemedicine was becoming more mainstream and was compensated now by Medicare and several private insurances. I considered working part time as a "tele-doctor", but again, I didn't need the money and I felt that what I really wanted was freedom to run my own schedule and not have to answer to a manager or a boss. I even considered volunteering at the county-sponsored free clinic for a day or two per month, but then decided that the type of patient I would be seeing there would not provide me with any of the satisfactions that I had found in private practice—long term relationship with patients—and would likely expose me to a segment of the local population that I did not want to assume medical liability for. In the end, I could not see any avenue for me to practice medicine in retirement. The good news was that I could tell my family, friends and neighbors that I was "retired" and not in the giving medical advice or prescriptions business any more. I could finally become a medical "lay-person", but give education and counsel when and if I decided to. I volunteered with my church to be a medical advisor to do screening reviews of potential missionary applicants. This allowed me the opportunity to keep my hand in medicine, but to do it at my own schedule. So, even now that I am retired, I am still "practicing medicine".

The political climate regarding health care in the United States became more rancorous during my retirement. Obamacare was a failure and a new

Republican president with a Republican majority congress was elected. But, although the push to "repeal and replace" Obamacare was all over the news, the new administration did not seem to be able to get the job done, and the proposed "replacement" for Obamacare is not a wholesale replacement but a series of "fixes" that in my view only served to make health care in the United States more insane and dysfunctional.   It was high political theater, but with no visible promise to actually make heath care in the US more available, sane or affordable. I was always a bit amused when the politicians and the news media talked about the citizens getting or being denied "health care" because they were not actually talking about doctors taking care of sick patients, but were talking about the structure and organization of paying for health care. That is the number one problem with the current health care discussion in the United States—it is not about optimizing the way that doctors take care of sick people, it is about paying for it. It is a political-economic football in a very high stakes game that the politicians are playing. In my view, this is just politics as usual with the big question being whether or not the United States is going to remain with a patchwork private pay/government pay system or go to a "single payer system" with the government assuming the control of the entire health care dollar. Almost certainly, in the end result, physicians will become employees of either big insurance companies or of the federal government. I see no joy in the practice of medicine in either scenario. The autonomy that was such a major attraction to the field of medicine in past generations will be dead and buried in another decade. It will be an entirely different demographic group of people with an entirely different work ethic and different work expectations that will populate the ranks of medical practitioners in the coming generation. Looking back, I clearly practiced medicine at the end of the "golden" era for the profession. Medicine may yet provide marvelous technological advances in the treatment of diseases, but it will lack the ability to inspire the passion and commitment that has been so characteristic of the medical practitioner in the past.

    I came from a family line that had no medical professionals in it. Other than for my son who is a nurse, I will leave no progeny to carry on in my place in this most honorable of professions.   In 20 years my family line will be no more educated or expert about medical issues than they would be if I had never been a practicing physician. I feel sorry for that. Not so much sorry for myself, but sorry for the fact that the current social climate has become toxic for the practitioners of medicine, and toxic to the patients who receive medical care. At a time when we stand on the technological and scientific threshold of a truly miraculous medical future we face having a medical system that is unfriendly—nay, toxic-- to the practitioners of the science and art of medicine. Will we fall victim to a dystopian system of medical care as portrayed in novels and movies where a highly technologically advanced but uncaring and unfeeling medical profession functions as an agent of the state (or of big-business)? I wish I could be more optimistic, but the current trend is not favorable.

Death and Taxes

So, I come to the end of my story about health care in America as I experienced it from the perspective of a physician. It has been a very eventful ride! The science of medicine has exploded with new understanding and treatments. The technology of medicine has produced miraculous machines that have advanced our ability to diagnose and treat disease. Medical insurance has become widespread if not universal but with it has come a mountainous burden of red tape and administrative bureaucracy. We are on the brink of being able to provide truly individualized medical care and at the same time on the brink of administratively mandated uniformity of care. Looking to the future I see more of the same—the good and the bad. Our population is outpacing our medical manpower's ability to serve their needs, and the costs of providing health care are becoming unsustainable. And in the face of all of this, the satisfaction of the providers of health care services is trending to an all-time low. Just when we are on the brink of a new miraculous era in medical treatments, the practitioners of medicine want to bail out and go and find a different line of work!

The purpose of health care is to promote optimum health and comfort for the American public with a minimum of cost. Health issues are very personal involving one person with problems that reduce their quantity and quality of life. When faced with a single patient, and taking no consideration for the greater society in which that patient lives the compassionate physician desires to do everything that is possible to help their patient. I still believe that at their core, most physicians desire to do the best for their patients…to "save their lives". When they are faced with a patient in pain, or suffering from any other medical problem the physician's first instinct is to make things better by the application of medical science and technology. In the intimate setting of this patient-physician interaction the costs of medical care are at most a distant secondary consideration. But knowing that medical care is expensive the responsible physician must also have an eye to the larger society and the costs of medical interventions. In an ideal world, the physician would be free to provide the best possible medical care to each individual patient with no regards to cost. We do not live in that ideal world! We as physicians are limited by two restraining considerations: (1) Death cannot be defeated, it can only be delayed; and (2) The costs of medical care quickly come to a point of diminishing returns where the application of additional medical care at an increasing cost make less and less of a difference. As the old adage goes: "there are only two things that are certain: death and taxes", and truly death and taxes define the practical limits of medical intervention. And yet, as a society we have not come to a reasoned, rational and unemotional conversation about these two restraining issues and instead we continue to push the limits of medical interventions with no serious thought given to how we will pay for them. There are even instances where patients and their advocates insist that new treatments that have not been fully tested and proven be available to them outside of the confines of a defined medical study of that treatment. What we have now is a dysfunctional system of paying for medical care that by itself leads to increases in spending with decreasing health outcomes per dollar spent. Physicians are tortured by this dysfunctional system and its unmanageable red tape and bureaucratic interference and are very dissatisfied with the present situation leading them to early retirement, burnout, and decreased job satisfaction. At a time of increasing medical technological "miracles" physicians are becoming less satisfied with their careers. Patients are increasingly tortured by this dysfunctional system by unequal access to quality medical care and by increasing out of pocket medical costs. It seems contrary to the concept of a compassionate society to have any one person forced into bankruptcy due to medical costs. It is contrary to good sense and public policy to bankrupt the economy to pay for medical costs. People should not have to choose between groceries and medical care. Our society as a whole is tortured by increasing public and government costs for paying the bill for medical care that is clearly now at crisis proportions. This crisis has led to a patchwork of ideas, programs, rules and regulations that have become impossible for physicians and patients to comply with, and which have not been demonstrated to fix the problem. Our current system (2017) is the most dysfunctional of the modern era.

It is time to stop this patchwork approach and to develop a unified, comprehensive and equally applied approach to the provision of medical care.

A component of a unified and consistent medical system will need to be a societal agreement on the topic of whether we are trying to extend life to its last possible day, or are we trying to manage the inevitable slide from independent life to dependency and subsequent death in the most compassionate and reasonable fashion. This is not a comfortable topic to think about, and it becomes less palatable when the discussion must lead to some public policy decisions. This decision must be made from a societal perspective since leaving it to an individual case by case decision process clearly increases the costs of providing the care, and the greater society is the entity that bears those costs. The question must be asked what is the primary value of medical care: the extension of life at any cost and with any degree of quality or the provision of care focused upon the quality of life with acceptance of our inevitable mortality? Who defines what "quality of life" means? And, how can we decide what constitutes quality of medical care delivered without a definition of what "quality of life" means? Shall we apply every available medical technology no matter how unlikely it is to extend life and return the patient to functional independence? Shall we withhold medical treatment in cases of medical futility? Who decides? And how do we define "futility" and who makes that definition?   What about the well described if uncommon "outliers" who recover with extraordinary medical care from an apparent terminal disease to have months or years of functional life? If we are going to allow for exceptions from the rules of treatment who makes those exceptions and who enforces them? These questions are embedded within our most deeply held and cherished American societal values and will not be easy to answer to everyone's satisfaction.

It seems obvious to me that we must move ahead to a "single payer system"—i.e. a nationalized health care system. The current patchwork of private and government insurance is torturing every single player in the health care arena. Politics with its competing philosophies and perverse motives has chosen health care as the political football in a high stakes game with the losers being the American public. I have not come to this conclusion willingly. It has always been my opinion and observation that the government is a terrible manager of the public's money. Speaking with some hyperbole it looks to me like for every $100 we tax payers give Washington the American public gets back $1 in benefit. And yet, I have even less faith that a single payer system managed by a private entity could do the job. The profit motive of private business is not compatible with the provision of compassionate and comprehensive medical care. Government management of the medical-industrial complex is in large part the root cause of the mess that we are in now! For every new health care rule passed by congress and administered by some government bureaucracy (and usually lobbied for by some well-funded special health care interest group) adept managers and lawyers find a way to modify their part of health care to the greatest personal financial advantage. To ask the American public to have faith that we can solve the financial crisis of health care in America just by passing some national health care legislation is to enter into the realm of fantasy! (The track record of ObamaCare is proof of that assertion.) But enter we must since continuing in the current system is worse than fantasy—it is the very definition of insanity!

So, what would the ideal national health care system look like? That is a question that will be debated for the next decade and the conclusion will be the subject of extreme political rancor. Hopefully though it will be a question that will be debated and not be like ObamaCare where Nancy Pelosi told the congress to "pass the legislation and then you can read it and see what it has in it" (that is not a direct quote but a paraphrase). This is too important for our nation and its people to be pushed upon us by political dictators and shaped by competing political ideologies. I also think that we cannot just pattern the coming US system after the Canadian system or the Norwegian system because our population is so much larger and more diverse than those countries and there is no evidence that their systems are scalable to the American public. No, we must craft a system with the American citizen in mind. I have no credentials to suggest that my ideas are the answer to the crisis, but I think that any new health care system we adopt in the US must address the following issues directly and with openness and forethought given to the consequences: (This list is not comprehensive and many other issues will be identified if enough forethought is given to crafting a new health care system.)

1. The cost of educating and training new physicians must be addressed. Since physicians are going to be paid less in the future under a national health care system the extremely high debt burden to obtain medical qualifications must be reduced. To not address this issue will transition our physician work force to imported foreign born persons, and increase the amount of health care delivered by non-physician practitioners—NPs and PAs.
2. Some national planning will be needed to be sure that our physician workforce is balanced to produce the proper number and proportion of primary care and specialty care physicians. This may curtail one of our deepest held cultural values—personal choice in deciding "what you want to be". Incentives such as debt forgiveness programs may need to be instituted to promote the needed specialties. Restriction of the numbers of the various post-graduate training opportunities may be needed. These measures will not be popular and may reduce the number of applicants for medical training.
3. Emphasis needs to be made to the US public in an effective manner to promote healthy life style choices. "Preventive" health care is not something that physicians practice, it is something that patients do. The incentive to choose healthy life style behaviors needs to be placed on the people who need to make the choice and not upon the medical practitioner. This issue and the following issue represent the greatest opportunities to significantly reduce the cost of a national health care system.
4. The unsupportable number of administrative jobs in health care will need to be severely reduced. This is contrary however to the manner of government behavior. If this is not done the new system will fail because of unaffordable expense. The single largest opportunity to reduce the cost of health care in America is to reduce the administrative burden.
5. We must find a balance between paying for necessary care and excluding payment for futile care. Rather than excluding payment for futile care, we must stop providing futile care. If individual patients insist upon futile care, it

should be at their own expense and not funded by the health insurance program.
6. We must extend coverage and benefits for managing the end of life.
7. We must allow some provision for private payment for extraordinary care to individuals who consider themselves to be outliers on the "futile care" definition. The cost of "futile care" must be privately borne.
8. We must modify tort laws to reflect a changed definition of what represents the standard of care. Quality of care definitions must be based upon an agreement of what represents quality of life. We will need to address whether or not the government can be held responsible for malpractice in a system where all physicians are employees of the government.
9. We must protect the status of physicians with MD degrees from encroachment upon their professional prerogatives by non-MDs. To do otherwise will result in the reduction of persons who pursue medical training and will further increase the proportion of foreign born and educated physicians in the US. It will also increase the proportion of medical care provided by less qualified practitioners such as PA's and NPs.
10. We must protect the prerogative of physicians to be the ones who define what represents quality medical care and not shift that decision to non-physician bureaucrats or politicians. Standards of care must be physician defined and not be allowed to be defined by legislatures or judges.
11. We must adopt a single, workable medical records system—an EHR—that allows for free flow of medical information and standardization of medical record keeping. Physician input into its design and function is essential or it will fail to provide its potential benefits. Stronger protections for digital record privacy will need to be crafted to protect patients.
12. We must insist that pharmaceuticals be priced comparatively from nation to nation and from region to region. The same is true for medical equipment and medical supplies. Negotiating prices for pharmaceuticals must be part of any program to reduce medical costs. The US cannot subsidize the pharmaceutical industry by paying higher prices for drugs than other countries do.

Epilogue

"So, Kirk", how was your experience being a doctor for the last 4 decades? That is a question I expect to have to answer more and more now that I am retired. Well, the answer is hard to get my hands and mind around to tell the truth! I found myself well suited by temperament and intellect to practice my specialty of internal medicine. I cared for my patients as I got to know them and still miss that close association that comes with a primary care specialty practice. I still have frequent dreams of being in the office or hospital working through patient care scenarios. Some of these dreams are pleasant, most are just very fatiguing, and some are nightmares! Such was the practice of medicine. I witnessed the advancement of the science and technology of medicine that in retrospect was breathtaking. But at the same time, I found that for any one patient it was a very short distance from initial symptoms to diagnosis to application of all that medicine had to offer. The therapeutic arsenal that we have as doctors is much broader than in the past but only a little deeper. We have many more treatment choices available but death still wins every time. Chronic disease management has become the most important medical task of our time. Disease management is the bedrock of medical practice. Headline grabbing technological advances in providing procedural medicine gets all the glory, but the chronic management of life long disease is where the health care system will win or lose both fiscally as well as in the health and "wellness" of the American public.

And, as a last word, would I advise my children or grandchildren to enter the medical profession? For now, I must sadly answer no! The current dysfunctional system with its ever-changing rules and no blue print for a better future is just too stressful a profession to subject my loved ones to. The politics of government and private insurance make the prospects for a happy result from the next changes to come unlikely. The physician is subject to such a long lineup of guidelines, requirements, incentives, risks, and uncertainties with managers of every kind looking over their shoulder and enforcing those rules with dictatorial techniques that finding joy in the profession is not possible. This is very sad commentary! The profession of medicine is capable of being the supreme service profession but is hindered by so much political, governmental and private interference that instead it has become the worst possible place for the altruistic minded person to labor. The practice of medicine requires compassion, altruism, and self-sacrifice but the current milieu offers no support or incentive to nurture those qualities. Until that situation changes I would be hesitant to recommend medicine as a career choice for anyone I know and care about. As I have said before, we stand at a time in history when the realities of "miracle" medical technologies are before us and yet the satisfaction that physicians feel from their work is surely near its lowest point of the modern era. At these crossroads must enter the physicians for the next generation. I wish them well. I am glad that I am not one of them.

About the Author

Dr. Anderson was born and grew up in Utah. He attended Brigham Young University and received a B.S. degree in Sociology with a minor in Psychology. Thereafter he attended medical school at the University of Utah graduating in 1977. His post-graduate training in internal medicine was at LDS Hospital in Salt Lake City, Utah. He entered private practice in 1980 with a small internal medicine clinic in Provo, Utah that grew to be the largest physician owned and operated medical practice in the State of Utah and practiced in that clinic for 35 years. He had a busy and active medical practice that included both clinic office practice and hospital care. Over the years he served in many hospital leadership roles including chairman of the Internal medicine department at two different hospitals, director of the hospital intermediate care unit, co-director of the hospital drug treatment program, chairman of the medical staff, and medical director. He also served on the board of directors of the medical group which he first joined in 1980 that grew from a small group of seven internists to over 150 multi-specialty physicians. He served as the primary care physician for his patients as well as a hospital consultant to many other physicians on the care of their patients.

Dr. Anderson is married to his wife Laura Lee since 1971 and together they have eight children, 15 grandchildren, three horses and two grand-dogs. In his free time, he fancies himself as a horseman and enjoys horseback riding throughout the intermountain west. He also had some limited experience as a horse "wrangler" for some small independent movies. He is now retired and trying to figure out what to do with this next chapter of his life.

www.ingramcontent.com/pod-product-compliance
Lightning Source LLC
Chambersburg PA
CBHW070242190526
45169CB00001B/279